XANDRIA WILLIAMS

VITAL SIGNS FOR CANCER

Protect yourself
from the onset or
recurrence of cancer

piatkus

PIATKUS

First published in Great Britain in 2010 by Piatkus

A CIP catalogue record for this book
is available from the British Library.

ISBN 978-0-7499-5247-1

Text design by Sam Charrington Design
Typeset in Utopia by M Rules
Printed and bound in Great Britain by
MPG Books, Bodmin, Cornwall

Papers used by Piatkus are natural, renewable and
recyclable products sourced from well-managed forests and certified
in accordance with the rules of the Forest Stewardship Council.

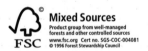

Mixed Sources
Product group from well-managed
forests and other controlled sources
www.fsc.org Cert no. SGS-COC-004081
© 1996 Forest Stewardship Council
FSC

Piatkus
An imprint of
Little, Brown Book Group
100 Victoria Embankment
London EC4Y 0DY

An Hachette UK Company
www.hachette.co.uk

www.piatkus.co.uk

I would like to dedicate this book to all those who have

- the courage to step beyond the medical model and look to the CAM therapies in their fight against cancer;
- the wisdom to recognise the power of prevention and the value of the tests for Vital Signs, described here;
- the commitment to follow through on what they learn; and
- the discipline needed to make the appropriate permanent and positive changes to their lifestyle.

Acknowledgements

Heartfelt thanks go to my agent, Sara Menguc, for her unstinting support in this project, in which she has been more than usually involved.

I have, as always, drawn on what I have learnt from the many thousands of patients and students with whom I have worked over the years; to them, too, I give thanks for their trust and for all they have done and shared.

My thanks also go to the team at Piatkus who have recognised the importance of this approach to cancer.

Contents

APPENDICES

Introduction and General Concepts

Vital Signs for Cancer is about the vital or important signs that can alert you to the possibility that you might be heading for degenerative diseases in general and cancer in particular. The Vital Signs may be symptoms that you can detect and, with the help given here, correct for yourself, or they may come in the form of the results of the many tests that are recommended in this book.

Cancer is a process that starts off with poor diet, poor nutrition, the presence of toxins, and seemingly minor problems with a number of aspects of your general health. Then, usually after many years, although sometimes much more rapidly, these signs cross the boundary and first individual cancer cells are formed and then a detectable tumour. In *Vital Signs for Cancer* you will learn how you can detect any of these early warning signs; you will learn about tests you can do and ways you can make the appropriate corrections.

Prevention is much easier than treatment. A benefit of using CAM (complementary, alternative and metabolic) therapies, however, is that the two often overlap. All of the suggestions made in this book for preventing cancer are also a vital part of your basic approach to treatment if you do have cancer, although then, of course, more is needed – much more.

The main thrust of this book is about the tests you can carry out; however, you will also find indications as to how to correct some of the problems. If the problems are simple, or if the indicated test result comes with its own suggestions for correction procedures, you can do a lot for yourself. You can, for instance, make appropriate dietary changes and follow some of the detox procedures.

Even when a practitioner is involved, the more you know about what you are being asked to do the better. You are more likely to comply with the suggestions you receive and to interpret and apply them correctly and in a positive frame of mind.

The detail

The topics covered in this book are necessarily broad and far ranging, and underlying them all is a great deal of theory and technical detail. Extensive explanation of all these terms would take the book to an unmanageable size. For this reason I have added an extensive Glossary at the end, and this should be your first port of call if you come to a term that you do not understand. If you still need further explanation, or the term you are looking for is not in the Glossary, an Internet search will generally provide a quick and simple explanation.

What You Will Find Inside

I have made a number of suggestions for supplements, specific foods and remedies. In general they are available from health-foods stores. Some, such as therapeutic coffee, are available from the sources listed in the Resources section at the back of the book.

I suggest many tests throughout the book. There are a few you can do yourself and these will be obvious as you work through, such as the 'spitting' test for *Candida albicans*. In general, however, the tests are carried out in several different laboratories, and you will find a list of these in Resources. Some of the laboratories are willing to take calls directly from individuals; however, they usually require a practitioner, be it a CAM therapist or a medical doctor, to make a formal request for the tests. Such a professional will also be required to help you interpret the results. Most of the laboratories indicated cover a wide and varying range of tests, so no attempt has been made here to list them, but a quick enquiry from you or your practitioner will soon find a laboratory that does the tests that interest you. Where a laboratory carries out one or two specialised tests these have been indicated but, by the time you are reading this book, these laboratories may be doing more. There are, of course, other laboratories in various parts of the UK and other countries, but local enquiries should enable you to find them.

The majority of the suggested tests are done using saliva, the breath, hair, urine or faeces, all of which are samples that can readily be sent by post, so the laboratory does not have to be close to you. Blood samples usually, but not always, need to arrive at the laboratory within one or two days, and this can generally be arranged via the postal service or courier companies. The laboratories will generally post out the appropriate sample kit with instructions as well as price details.

You will notice that I refer to 'optimising strategies' where you might expect to find the word 'treatments'. I have done this to avoid making claims – actions that are often frowned upon, particularly in relation to cancer.

If you are concerned about preventing or treating cancer and you are looking for a CAM practitioner that specialises in this, you may be surprised to find how difficult your search can become. That is because, in the UK, no one is allowed to claim or advertise that they treat cancer (British Cancer Act of 1939, plus developing legislation from European authorities). You will find advertisements by CAM practitioners who will help you if you have arthritis, allergies, weight problems or digestive upsets, but not if you have or are concerned about cancer. One of the reasons for writing this book is so that you know what is important and can use this as a guide when looking for a practitioner to help you with your prevention programme.

If you are looking for a CAM practitioner and want a way to assess the extent to which they can help you, then check them out against this book. Make sure that they understand the concepts discussed here and recognise their relevance to the start of the cancer process. Make sure that they know about, and can help you with, the CA Profile test, described later, which can give you the earliest possible sign that you might already be heading for cancer.

Finally, a word about solid-tumour cancers versus blood-related cancers. By far the majority of cancers involve solid tumours. It is true that modern medicine has had some significant success in treating some of the blood-related cancers, but almost negligible success in treating solid-tumour cancers. In much of the following discussion reference is made, on several occasions, to the tumour aspect of cancer. It should not be assumed from this that the ideas expressed here will not help you to prevent the blood cancers. The general ideas apply to all and can be used in relation to the prevention of all types of cancer or in partnership with your own, possibly medical, therapies for any type of cancer.

I hope you will find this book helpful towards understanding the Vital Signs that can lead to cancer and how you might be able to act early so that you will at least halt their further development.

Xandria Williams

PART 1
A NEW APPROACH TO CANCER

CHAPTER 1

Overview

Cancer is unique among health problems. In heart disease it is your heart and arteries that are unhealthy and need to be treated; their structure and function need to be corrected. In asthma it is your lungs and bronchial tubes that are unhealthy and need to be treated. In diabetes it is your management of your blood glucose level that is faulty, and your cellular response to insulin has to be corrected. In indigestion the function of your digestive system needs to be corrected. In osteoporosis it is your bones that are not healthy and their structure that needs to be corrected.

Cancer is different. It is not a disease of a single organ or system. You do not have prostate cancer because your prostate is not doing its job properly, or breast cancer because your breasts are not fulfilling their function. In cancer you do not have a disease *of* an organ or system, you have a disease *in* an organ or system.

It is very important to understand this when it comes to both prevention and recovery. You can prevent heart problems by appropriate dietary modifications that benefit your heart and arteries. You can prevent asthma by avoiding allergens and supplying the nutrients needed by your bronchial muscles. You can prevent diabetes by removing sugar and refined carbohydrates from your diet and ensuring an adequate supply of chromium, vanadium and related trace nutrients. You can prevent digestive problems by relaxing while you eat, eating correctly, and avoiding allergens and toxins. You can prevent osteoporosis by ensuring an adequate intake of the appropriate minerals needed by your bones and by doing regular exercise.

These are, of course, very much simplified suggestions, and a lot more can be done, and may need to be done, in the treatment of the health problems mentioned, and of others. However, the common denominator in all of these problems is that the solution is aimed at improving the structure or function of the organ or tissue that is faulty.

When you think in terms of treating cancer, you do not in general think of treating the organ in which the cancer is situated. You do not aim to improve the function of your ovaries or uterus if you have ovarian or uterine cancer. You do not aim to improve the function of your kidneys if you have kidney cancer, or of your lungs if you have lung cancer.

So what do you do, and on what basis? This is where the two types of health care, practised today, divide. We have the establishment approach that focuses almost entirely on the use of medical drugs and surgery. We can call this the medical–drug–surgery or MDS approach. We have the natural-therapies approach, in the broadest meaning of the words, which is based on an understanding of human metabolism, nutrition, herbal medicine, homoeopathy, structural therapies, such as chiropractic and osteopathy, and different forms of energy medicine. Much of it is based on a clear understanding of the biochemistry and metabolic pathways in the body and their correction. This is variously referred to as alternative medicine or complementary medicine. We can call this the complementary, alternative and metabolic, or the CAM, approach.

In the MDS approach, cancer is identified by the presence of a tumour or, as in the case of blood cancers or early cervical cancer, by the presence of transformed, altered or faulty cells. It is a localised problem, in the tissue in which the tumour or altered cells are found. In this approach the treatment is aimed almost totally at eradicating these cells or destroying the tumour. Once the tumour has been removed, or if it is thought that all the cells have been destroyed, or if the surgeon 'got it all', the problem is deemed largely to have been solved. Little thought is given to the reasons why it started and, therefore, how a recurrence can be prevented.

In the CAM approach, cancer is recognised as being a systemic problem that affects the whole body. CAM therapists are used to taking this view. They are familiar with working with the whole person, not just the organ or system that is faulty. Therefore, the help they offer someone with cancer will be systemic rather than aimed specifically at the tumour. This is the approach taken in this book.

I propose an extension of this view of cancer. I suggest that cancer is a process, the cancer process, in which the transformed cells, or the tumour, are merely the final outcome. This cancer process occurs in two phases. In Phase One you do not yet have, and may never have, cancer, but you are moving along a progression of health disorders, or predisposing factors, that progressively and cumulatively increase your likelihood of entering Phase Two. Phase Two starts when the first permanent transformed or cancerous cells form and are not destroyed by your defences. This Phase can be detected by a test you will learn about that is thought to show up a positive result within six to eight weeks of the formation of these early cells, and possibly as much as 10 to 12 years before a tumour has grown to a detectable size. If you are impatient to know more about this test you can leap forward to Chapter 7, but I suggest it is more helpful to read your way towards that.

There is power behind this concept of cancer. Firstly, once you understand that the predisposing factors of Phase One lead towards Phase Two, you can contribute to the prevention of cancer by correcting or minimising all the predisposing factors that may apply to you. Secondly, if you have had cancer in the past, you can greatly reduce your risk of having either a recurrence of the old cancer or of developing a new cancer by applying this same strategy. Thirdly, if you currently have cancer, you can apply the same philosophy to utilising these strategies to support whatever therapy you are undergoing. It will help to prevent all the micro recurrences that are going on daily until such time as your cancer is brought under control by your chosen therapies.

Why I Chose Naturopathy

I am a scientist, I have always been a scientist. At five years of age I loved arithmetic, then it was general science. Arithmetic got even better when it expanded into mathematics. General science got even better when it was subdivided and I discovered chemistry. My first decade after graduation from the chemistry department at Imperial College in London was spent in the mining industry as a geochemist involved in mineral exploration. This had little to do with human health, yet even then it made no sense to me for medicine to focus on treating disease when it would be better to focus on preventing it. Nor did it make much sense to me, when considering ill-health problems, to place the primary focus on a bewildering array of drugs, all of which had toxic side effects. Surely, I thought even then, the first aim should be to assist the body to repair itself. I have continued to think so ever since.

Soon after I turned 30 I swapped professions and changed from geochemistry to biochemistry, which I have loved ever since. I taught biochemistry and nutrition in chiropractic and naturopathic colleges in Sydney, Australia for nearly 20 years. Naturopathy and the detailed biochemistry of the body, our food and human health so intrigued me that I did the full three-year naturopathic course and have been in private practice for the last three decades or more.

As soon as I discovered naturopathy it was immediately and abundantly clear that the naturopathic philosophy and my own philosophy were essentially the same:

- First, do no harm.
- Give the body all the nutrients it needs to function to its best.
- Remove all toxins that interfere with normal and healthy metabolism.
- Work with the whole body and its fundamental metabolism.
- Think of the symptoms as a guide to underlying problems, not as the problems themselves.
- Symptoms and problems should be resolved and not suppressed.

Inevitably a number of people, right from the start of my naturopathic career, came to me with cancer and asked if I treated it. I don't treat cancer. No naturopath treats cancer. No good naturopath treats any named disease. By virtue of the philosophy briefly itemised above, we treat the whole person. Once you remove the roots of the weeds, the flower heads and clinging vines will fall away and the garden's health will be restored.

In the 1980s, we could offer relatively little to the person suffering from cancer, yet in spite of this we had some noticeable success, including my own first patient with cancer, Malcolm I., who you will learn about later. Our knowledge and our treatment options have expanded almost exponentially since then. Today the natural therapies have a lot to offer the person wanting to avoid cancer, avoid a recurrence or help themselves through the process of overcoming cancer.

During the past decade I have become progressively more and more interested in cancer and the CAM or naturopathic approach to supporting people who have it. As soon as I started this line of in-depth research it became clear that the intervening years had been enormously productive. We have come to a much better understanding, from a metabolic perspective, of the causes of cancer. We have developed a greater understanding of the predisposing factors, and what it is, biochemically, that triggers the final tip over from a toxic, damaged or deranged cell to a cancer cell. As a result, we have developed some powerful tools for preventing cancer and for supporting people when they are undergoing treatment for cancer.

How modern medicine contrasts with naturopathy

Modern medicine, the MDS approach, offers little in the way of prevention. Although it has had some notable successes with some of the blood cancers, it has achieved relatively little in the treatment of solid tumour cancers, when the hype and the smudging of statistics is set aside.

Some sobering figures come from a recently published book in the US.[1] The cost of cancer drugs, worldwide, is US $40 billion per year, second only to medications for heart problems, but rising at double the annual growth rate. This is despite the fact that 'in most [non-blood cancers] chemotherapy is remarkably ineffective'.

A study of American and Australian data has shown that the survival rate is 63 per cent, but that chemotherapy contributes only 2 per cent to this. It showed zero effect on multiple myeloma, soft-tissue sarcomas, melanoma of the skin, cancer of the bladder, kidney, pancreas, prostate and uterus.

Two examples are given: lung cancer kills 150,000 Americans a year, costs US $40,000 per person and treatment extends a person's life on average by two months (plus the cost of the side effects, which can be brutal). For metastatic breast cancer the figure was US $360,000 per person.

The economics are disturbing on another front. The authors state that oncologists are among the highest paid doctors, their salaries are increasing faster than those of any other specialists and more than 50 per cent of their income comes from selling cancer drugs. Yet, 'The age-adjusted mortality rate for cancer is essentially unchanged over the past half-century.' This is in spite of the huge increase in funding and research during that same time.[2]

In another report chemotherapy has been shown to increase the five-year survival rate by only 2.3 per cent (Australian figures) or 2.1 per cent (US figures).[3]

In contrast to the CAM approach, the MDS system:

- First, *does* do harm – there is no medical drug that does not have some harmful side, or toxic, effect.
- Largely ignores nutrition and the possibility of nutrient deficiencies, yet that is the fuel on which the body runs.
- Almost never incorporates any detox strategy in its treatment programmes, and often increases the body's toxic load, yet many of these toxins are carcinogens.

- Focuses on the symptom, not the whole body, hence we have specialists who focus only on the digestive tract, the heart, the kidneys, and so on.

- Frequently suppresses symptoms without correcting the underlying cause. Examples include the use of drugs to lower blood pressure, block out pain, block inflammation or suppress a temperature without correcting the cause. In fact a temperature is an essential part of boosting the immune system so that it can deal with the problem, as you will learn later, and it should not be suppressed.

The Focus of this Book

In this book I will be focusing on the three topics mentioned, on what you can do to:

1   Avoid cancer, if you have not developed it.
2   Avoid a recurrence, if you are in remission.
3   Assist the process of overcoming cancer, if you have been diagnosed with it.

You will learn about the important aspects of your diet and about nutrients, followed by a consideration of your delivery route or digestive system. We will discuss toxins and how to detect them, eliminate existing ones and avoid new ones. You will learn about a variety of predisposing factors, how to test for them and, if necessary, correct or remove them. You will learn about a number of tests you can do to both detect problems and then monitor your treatment of them as they are corrected.

Vital Signs for Cancer, the title of this book, was chosen for a number of reasons. Throughout the following pages, I refer to a number of tests that I encourage you to do. The results of these will give you vital information as to the state of your health. Almost certainly some of them will indicate problems or signs (the Vital Signs) that all is not as it should be if you wish to have maximum health. You should pay attention to these Vital Signs, or signals, and should act accordingly. This may mean changing your diet, adding supplements, going on a detox programme, reducing your level of stress, or correcting any one of the other predisposing factors that could, if a final trigger is applied, tip you over into the development of cancer – that could move you from Phase One to Phase Two of the cancer process.

This is a self-help book, not a do-it-yourself book. It is primarily a book about learning and testing. It is about the tests you can do, or can ask to have done, to find out if you have any problems. The aim is to encourage you to do these tests and to pay attention to, and to act on, the results. It is not primarily about treatments, as these will vary with your individual results and with the individual combination of results that you obtain. Inevitably, however, some optimising strategies will be indicated by the nature of your results and the discussions around them.

Remember, I use the term 'optimising strategies' rather than 'treatment' because it better describes what you are trying to do and because of the prohibition on claiming that anything helps to treat cancer. The emphasis here is on minimising metabolic errors, not on treating a disease. This is another reflection of the difference between CAM therapies and the MDS system.

In my next book, *Cancer Concerns,* you will find a discussion of Phase Two and optimising strategies for some of the more complex issues. This is a more technical book, aimed at people with some background knowledge or who, possibly through force of circumstances and necessity, have given themselves a crash course on learning more about cancer. There is a reason for this. I have learned over the years that people who take a serious interest in the prevention and, if appropriate, treatment of their cancer become very well informed about what is happening to them and how they can help themselves. They have many questions and they are looking for detailed explanations of what is happening, what is being suggested to them and how they can help themselves. Cancer is a serious, complex and controversial disease. Nonetheless, I have attempted to make this book as comprehensible as possible.

The Importance of Prevention

Prevention is very much easier than treatment. This is even more true of cancer than of most other health problems, and the subject is discussed in more detail in Chapter 5.

Prevention happens on a day-by-day basis, on a second-by-second basis, even on a micro-second-by-micro-second basis. So if you do currently have cancer, this book may also help you. By applying these prevention strategies you can help to stop each new individual cell that might otherwise turn into a cancer cell, or develop into an increasingly active cancer cell, from doing so. All these optimising strategies can help to rebuild your health. As such you can use them in combination with whatever therapy you choose to follow and improve your chance of recovery.

Although this book is primarily about prevention of cancer, in the process of doing this you will be rebuilding your health and thus inevitably you will also be preventing the occurrence of a number of other potential degenerative diseases. So this book can be for you even if you are not only, or primarily, concerned about cancer but just have a general desire to optimise your health.

It has frequently been stated that approximately two-thirds or 65 per cent of cancers are diet and lifestyle related. This is a figure that is commonly bandied about, without any real evidence-based suggestion as to the cause of the other 35 per cent. There are now suggestions that the figure is as high as, or possibly even higher than, 90 per cent[4] and that only 10 per cent or less of the incidence is genetic or viral related.

If diet and lifestyle play such an important role in the aetiology of the disease, then you are in a very powerful position. By changing your diet and lifestyle you have the potential to make a huge impact on your reduction of risk and the prevention of a possible cancer.

Cancer is a Process

The cancer process can be a lengthy one. It can last for many years until the final point, the discovery of a tumour, is reached.

Since no one is in absolutely perfect and total health right down to the cellular level, everyone can be considered to be in Phase One or, to put it another way, in the precancerous phase. It may seem strange to imply that if you do not have cancer you are in a precancerous stage. Current figures vary, depending on you source, from one in two men and one in three women, or approximately 40 per cent, and up to as high as 70 per cent for people born now. Taking the average you have a 50–50 chance of developing cancer. These are not great odds. When deaths are aggregated by age, cancer has surpassed heart disease as the leading cause of death for those younger than age 85 since 1999.[5] This being so, it behoves you to do as much as you possibly can to avoid cancer and to stop yourself from becoming one of the cancer statistics. It is better to think like this and to err on the side of over-caution than to put your head in the sand and simply hope that cancer will never happen to you.

You may be in reasonable health, you may even think of yourself as being totally healthy. Or you may have a variety of health problems, many or all of which may be predisposing you to developing cancer, if or when you are exposed to a final trigger large enough to convert healthy cells into cancerous ones.

Act Now

Keep in mind that within Phase One you do not have cancer, but as you move along it, as you acquire or develop progressively more and more of these predisposing factors, the odds on you developing cancer increase. All these predisposing factors are things you can remedy – and you can do so now, before you have cancer. Now, therefore, is the very best time to take action.

Phase Two starts with the first permanent cancer cells, and dealing with them is outside the scope of this book. However, it is worth noting that these early cancer cells may be present long before, possibly many years before, a tumour is large enough to be detected, even if you knew exactly where to look for it, and certainly long before the tumour is of a significant size to lead to symptoms that would alert you to its possible presence.

Modern medicine does not, in most cases, detect or diagnose solid-tumour cancers, which are by far the most common, until there is a tumour large enough to cause symptoms, by which time it can be many centimetres in size. Doctors then need to be able to feel or visually detect and measure it. This is too late for many therapies to be effective. The tests described in Chapter 7 will enable you to detect the very beginnings of cancer within about six weeks of the formation of the first cancer cells. Better still, this panel of tests assesses your whole body. There is no need for a lot of separate tests to check for all the different possible cancer locations. The results, if outside of the normal ranges, will alert you to the need to deal with these predisposing factors even more aggressively and to explore further ways of stopping the cancer process.

It is very much easier to reverse out of deteriorating health before cancer develops than if you wait until a significant tumour is detected. Equally, it is very much easier to deal with precancerous cells, or very early cancer, if you do detect it, than with a fully developed tumour.

Finally, if you do have cancer, eliminating the predisposing factors discussed here should be a major part of your recovery plan and will greatly increase your chances of returning to full health, whether you choose to use conventional medical treatments or alternative strategies.

You will learn:

- How to take better care of your health.
- How to avoid the predisposing factors.
- How to reduce your risk of developing cancer, significantly, if you do not already have it.
- How to detect it long before a tumour has fully developed, at a stage when you have a very good chance of success.
- How, if you are in remission, to remain there and avoid a recurrence.
- How you can improve your chance of recovery if you already have a malignant tumour.

Over the past 30-plus years in practice I have seen countless people and observed the progression of their health. Some have attended to minor health problems, focused on prevention and remained well for decades. Others have said 'it is not too bad, I can put up with it' or for some other reason chosen not to improve their lifestyle or correct the minor problems. These people have commonly moved from mild ill health, through a variety of stages, to such degenerative diseases as arthritis, diabetes, heart disease and cancer. Once these diseases occur there is often the wish expressed that they had paid more attention, and taken corrective measures, sooner. It is in the hope that you will be, or can be encouraged to be, one of the former group that this book is written. Health often seems to be the prerogative of youth. Yet countless times, when people have been willing to make appropriate changes, I have seen them reverse out of the various degenerative diseases, back to greatly improved, if not perfect, health. It is almost never too late, although the later you leave it the more difficult it becomes.

Rosie S

Rosie told me that her mother had started to develop arthritis in her early fifties and been crippled into immobility by 70. Rosie was 52 and beginning to feel the symptoms. By changing her diet, and taking the appropriate supplements, we achieved a state whereby she became and remained pain-free, and remained essentially so into her eighties. She did become stiff but very much less so than her mother. The prevention of one degenerative disease is often thought to lead to the prevention of others.

CHAPTER 2

An Alternative Approach

Cancer is the greatest health fear in the minds of most people. It may even be more feared than heart disease, terrorism or senility. It is so feared that, all too often, people are unwilling to test for any early warning signs – the Vital Signs we will be talking about here – knowing, or assuming, that if positive signs suggestive of cancer are found they will be subjected to a barrage of unpleasant medical procedures with little hope of a successful outcome. You will learn, in the following pages, that there is much that you can do to avoid cancer and, if the early warning signs are there, there is a great deal you can do to help reverse the process before a tumour forms.

Do you have cancer? Have you had cancer? If so, you are not alone. According to Cancer Research UK, there are approximately 289,000 new cases of cancer diagnosed each year in the UK. That means that someone is diagnosed with cancer every two minutes, day and night, 365 days a year. The statistics vary with the source, but you have a greater than 35 per cent chance of developing cancer at some time in your life, and the risk is rising (see page 14). The incidence of cancer has increased by 25 per cent since 1975. About 75 per cent of cases occur in people aged 60 and over. Around 1 per cent of cancers occur in children, teenagers and young adults. However, children who survive cancer have a greater risk of another cancer later in life than children who have not had cancer. The most common forms of cancer are breast, lung, bowel and prostate, and these together account for over half of all new cancers each year.[6]

According to US figures made available in 2007, cancer now happens to approximately 50 per cent of men and approximately 35 per cent of women. In a June 2009 statement the M. D. Anderson Cancer Center in the US forecast that, on present indications, the number of new cancer cases diagnosed each year in the US will increase by 45 per cent over the next 20 years. Even more alarmingly, they anticipate that there will be significant increases in high mortality cancers such as those of the liver, pancreas and stomach.[7]

Cancer is one of the most preventable diseases. Remember, given that the majority of cancers are caused by faulty diet and lifestyle, and environmental factors, this prevention is largely within your own control. You may not be able to change everything about your environment, but you can do a great deal and you can certainly improve your diet and change many harmful aspects of your lifestyle. Thus you can improve your overall health and increase your ability to protect yourself from much of what you cannot change. In this book you will learn how.

There are many strategies you can use to reverse both phases of the cancer process, and the sooner you start adopting these strategies the healthier you can be and the greater your chance of avoiding cancer, recovering from it, or preventing a recurrence.

How Common is Cancer and How Successful is the MDS System at Treating It?

There have been many claims that we are 'winning the war against cancer'. But are we?

A lot has to do with what is given on the death certificate as to the cause of death. Someone might have cancer and then get pneumonia. Either could be noted as their cause of death. If you want to 'improve' the cancer survival figures, you would put pneumonia as the cause of death. There are almost certainly many more deaths from cancer than are actually recorded, for this reason.

Survival statistics depend on what you call cancer and how you define a 'cure'. There was a jump in the recovery or survival figures when skin cancers were added to the total, since few people die from skin cancers (excluding melanomas). The figures also improved in America when they excluded black Americans, who have a lower survival rate than white Americans.

In relation to cancer (but to no other health problem) survival is generally considered to mean that the person has survived for more than five years from diagnosis. You may still have cancer, you may die a few days later, but if you live for five years you enter the statistics as 'cured'. There has been talk of redefining 'cured' as having survived for a shorter period than five years after diagnosis. This, if it occurs, will seem to improve the survival figures but would have no bearing on the true state.

We are told that early detection of a tumour improves survival, but is this true? With early detection you may simply know about it for longer but still die at the same time. If someone's early detection is day one and they live for five years and a week, they are defined as cured. If it was detected later, say a year later, on day 367, they have only survived another four years since diagnosis and so have been defined as not cured. Early detection only *seems* to have increased their survival time and improved the cure rate. All that has really happened is that the person has known about it for longer. Early detection of a tumour is very different from early detection of Phase One of the cancer process. If you can detect the latter and make appropriate corrections, as is discussed in this book, you can greatly increase your chances of avoiding the development of Phase Two and a tumour.

A lot more could be said about the politics behind cancer claims, but that is not the purpose of this book. It is important, however, that you recognise that, in spite of the great 'war on cancer', there has been neg-ligible improvement in the medical treatment of, and recovery from, cancer in the past 50 years,[8] and there has been a significant increase in its rate of occurrence. For all these reasons, and more, we need to put greater emphasis on prevention, and this prevention should be targeted, monitored and made as effective as possible. Complacency is inappro-priate.

Another reason for giving you the above information is to encourage you not to put all your eggs in one basket. The MDS system has little to offer you in the way of sound and effective prevention strategies. It may help you if you already have a cancer, but even then there is so much more you can and should do by incorporating into your strategy all that you will learn here. Why hop on one leg when you can run on two?

Start at the Beginning, Not at the End

Because cancer is a process and not simply the presence of a tumour, it follows that you cannot cure cancer and prevent its recurrence by simply attacking the end result, the tumour. A tumour does not suddenly appear, fully formed. It is the result of the activities that occur within Phase Two of the cancer process. As Phase Two starts with the first cell that 'goes wrong', if you could detect this first error of your metabolism you could stop and reverse the process right at the start.

Unfortunately, the medical profession relies on detecting a fully formed tumour before a diagnosis of cancer is made, and by this time, with the best equipment available, it will already be at least few millimetres in size and consist of billions of cells. It may well be very much bigger. Many patients present with a problem that turns out to be related to one or more tumours of many centimetres in size. When these are detected this late, recovery is all the more difficult.

To ensure prolonged recovery from cancer you must do more than get rid of the tumour. You have to reverse Phase Two of the cancer process and eliminate the predisposing factors of Phase One. Once you understand *how* you have developed cancer you can work *with* your body, not *against* it, to ensure optimal long-term health and the prevention of a recurrence.

Surgery, chemotherapy and radiation are all aimed simply at destroying the tumour. They do nothing to reverse the cancer process. They work against the tumour but they also, in many respects, work against your body. The hope is that your body can better withstand the destructive treatment that is applied than can the cancer cells.

Many of the chemotherapy drugs work against rapidly dividing cells. Unfortunately for your body, this includes the cells lining your digestive tract as well as your hair cells. Thus, your delivery route for nutrients is compromised. Many chemotherapy agents work best in oxygen-rich cells; these are your healthy cells, not your cancer cells, which tend to be oxygen deficient or anaerobic cells.

For these and many other, similar, reasons, it is no wonder that the 'war on cancer' has not, in spite of the billions of pounds or dollars that have been thrown at it, achieved a significant improvement in benefit over the past decades since the 'war' was initiated.

The CAM Difference

If you implement what you will learn in the following pages, you will be working *with* your body and drawing on an invaluable support system.

While you do all this you will achieve a number of other health benefits as positive spin-offs:

- Your overall health will improve as you improve your health from the cells up.
- You will have more energy and an increased sense of well-being as you improve the metabolism within your cells.
- Your confidence will increase as you use the tests that are described and learn just which avenues you need to follow to accomplish these goals.
- You will gain peace of mind as you are able to monitor your progress and be sure that you are not slipping backwards.

All you need is the commitment, the willpower and the discipline to do what is required. However, this is a very big 'all' and not everyone is willing to make such a commitment. If you are, be ready to make some major changes in your life, but be prepared too for some very exciting and positive results.

Cancer is a serious problem, and no one has all the answers. The following cannot be over-emphasised: you should find yourself a practitioner whom you like, can trust, feel comfortable with and who understands the way you want to work. If the ideas expressed in this book make sense to you, then make sure your practitioner is familiar with them. This practitioner can be a CAM therapist or a medical practitioner who has also chosen to incorporate the CAM concept into their treatment protocols. If your aim is to avoid cancer, you will almost certainly do best with a CAM practitioner. If you have cancer, you may want to work with someone with a variety of skills. The important thing is to find someone who can cover a number of approaches, including those described in the following pages, and who can work with whatever other therapies you choose to use.

Finding such a person is not always easy

Remember, finding a CAM practitioner is made more difficult by the legal restrictions placed on people working in this field. This means that once you have cancer you are at a disadvantage when compared to having any other health problem. Be prepared to put some additional effort into this at the start. Remember that in the UK there are serious rules against anyone who wants to let it be known that they treat cancer. Naturopaths or CAM therapists are allowed to state that they work with the whole body (which is, of course, precisely what they do want to do) but are not allowed to claim that they 'treat cancer'. If you understand this, you may better understand why, for instance, you cannot readily find a list of CAM therapists who work with people who have cancer.

You will also understand their underlying meaning when they say things like, 'I can help with your overall health, but I don't "treat cancer" as such.' And, after all, it is your 'overall health' that you want to correct, for by doing that, having cancer will be impossible.

When you find someone who meets the criteria in this book, stick with them, even when they make some major demands of you. It is often tempting to find a practitioner who offers you an easy route, but they will rarely be as successful. If you have cancer, you have a major challenge on your hands and you need, and will benefit from, all the help you can get, and all the positive changes you can make. Equally, you cannot simply rely on books, however helpful they may be. Find yourself a practitioner.

Above all, find yourself a practitioner who understands the cancer process as discussed in the next chapter.

CHAPTER 3

The Cancer Process

Let's imagine a fairly typical example of someone going through life until, finally, they develop a tumour.

A Child is Born, and Life Begins

In our scenario, the individual is born healthy. If they are lucky they are breastfed. This gives their immune system the best chance to develop fully as they absorb all the immune factors from their mother's milk. It also means that their digestive tract is not challenged by foreign foods, particularly foreign proteins, during the first few months of life. If they are not breastfed they already start off at a disadvantage.

Once weaned, however, their problems generally start. They are probably fed pasteurised and homogenised dairy products (which contain damaged proteins and damaged or lost nutrients), white bread, flour and rice (which are vitamin and mineral deficient and lacking in fibre), sugar (which lacks any beneficial nutrients and challenges the pancreas and its insulin production), overheated fats (these develop toxic compounds, such as malondialdehyde, the dangerous and carcinogenic trans-fatty acids, and free radicals such as reactive oxygen species). They take in a vast array of food additives in the form of colours, preservatives, emulsifiers, stabilisers, homogenisers and artificial flavours, plus a range of hormones, growth factors and antibiotics found in animal products and agricultural chemicals such as pesticides and herbicides. They will live in a house where the usual chemical cleaners, bleaches, polishes, deodorisers, sanitisers, perfumed sprays, starching sprays, oven cleaners and other household chemicals are used, none of which are healthy. As they grow older, they then use a range of toiletries, cosmetics or after-shave lotions (depending on their gender).

As a child they are vaccinated. If or when they are sick they are given, or take, a variety of drugs, such as painkillers and antibiotics, possibly other specific and stronger drugs. As they grow up they drink alcohol, possibly to excess, and they might take drugs. They have (toxic) mercury fillings put into their teeth cavities and possibly implant a root canal (a dangerous focus for bacterial infections that are often asymptomatic). If they live in towns or cities they breathe in polluted air, if they live in the country they are subjected to the various sprays used in agricultural practices. Their body is bombarded by electromagnetic fields from radio, television, mobile phones, and many other sources, and by various sources of radioactive radiation. Their diet remains poor, lacking sufficient essential nutrients and laden with unwanted chemicals that benefit the food companies far more than the consumer.

As a result they become undernourished, at least in terms of nutrients, if not in terms of quantity, and overloaded with toxins. Many of the toxins are carcinogens, meaning they are capable of triggering the conversion of healthy cells into cancerous cells, either on their own or in combination with each other or with the various metabolic errors that can result from nutrient deficiencies.

Over the years their digestive system becomes compromised. If they eat a lot of sugar they may first become hypoglycaemic and then, in later years, diabetic. Their arteries clog up, their heart becomes stressed and blood pressure rises, but their circulation may be reduced. They work long hours, get into uncomfortable situations, are unhappy, angry, irritated or frustrated and stressed – all of which overtaxes their adrenal glands, which become exhausted.

Where Does this Lead?

All of the above occurs in Phase One of the cancer process, and contributes to a steady sequence of events and insults, all constituting predisposing factors that gradually weaken the person's health and make them more and more susceptible to cancer. 'They are all part of life', you may say. This is true, but if you want to live a long, healthy and cancer-free life you should make them as small a part of your life as possible.

Eventually, the final trigger comes that tips them over into Phase Two of the cancer process. It could be an increased exposure to any of the thousands of carcinogens to which they are subjected. It could be a significant stress that finally and completely exhausts their adrenal glands. It could be any one (or more) of a number of triggers that might not even be major in themselves but that have disastrous consequences when added to the existing predisposing factors.

After that happens they are in Phase Two of the cancer process, the phase when long-lived cancer cells become established, reproduce and multiply, out of control. From this point on in the developing cancer process there are cancer cells that are not being destroyed by their body's defence system. These may lie quietly for a while, possibly for a few years, and then be triggered into increased activity following further stimulation by more predisposing factors. This is why it is so important to test for, and correct, all predisposing factors and to do the CA Profile, which is described in Chapter 7. Otherwise, these cancer cells may multiply immediately, possibly silently, and constitute a fast-growing tumour.

———————————————

Before we can discuss alternative approaches to health care and to preventing serious health problems it would be helpful to define the concepts. So it is time to explain just what is meant by CAM therapies.

CHAPTER 4

What is CAM ?

In Australia, where I trained, the terms naturopath and naturopathy are well established and clearly understood. Naturopathy is recognised as an all-embracing natural therapy system. As far back as the late 1970s the naturopathic diploma was a three-and-a-half year full-time course, of over 3,000 in-college hours, covering all the Western-based natural therapies other than chiropractic and osteopathy. It included, and still includes, nutrition, herbal or botanical medicine, homoeopathy, massage and a number of other alternative therapies. Naturopathy in Australia and America is the major overarching natural medicine.

In the UK, the term 'naturopath' is less well known. People know of homoeopathy and some people train as nutritionists or herbalists. For a while, use was made of two terms, 'complementary medicine' and 'alternative medicine', both relating to the natural therapies by comparison with drug medicine. Neither of these terms on their own was deemed to be satisfactory and so the term CAM has evolved. For many it stands for complementary and alternative medicine, for others it is short for complementary, alternative and metabolic – a form I prefer, as 'CAM therapy' then includes an emphasis on restoring the individual's metabolism to normal. The term 'naturopath' is to me the more useful and appropriate, but I bow to local usage and have used the term 'CAM therapies' throughout this book.

The Evolution of Health Care

It is interesting to consider a very brief and simplified overview of the way health care has evolved through the millennia. In ancient times it was the wise men of the tribe, the witch doctors, who provided the ancient wisdoms and had the most dramatic effects on the health of the tribe. They healed the body and the spirit, often in dramatic ways. However, it was the women, working away quietly in the background, who came to understand the benefits of different foods, herbs and other plant and animal substances, as well as remedies in the treatment of day-to-day health problems. Over the centuries the witch doctors evolved and sub-divided into the church leaders on the one hand and the medical or drug doctors on the other, the latter being deemed, rightly or wrongly, to be technical, scientific, appropriate activities for men and worthy of respect. The women's role with nutrition and herbs evolved into nutrition and domestic science on the one hand, and health care using natural reme-dies on the other; both were considered 'soft' subjects, suitable, in a politically incorrect age of macho superiority, for women. This in part explains the placing of drug medicine in the universities and the CAM therapies on the outer edge in colleges that are only gradually becoming recognised within the educational system.

When Two Views Coincide

There is another aspect to this history and it concerns two Frenchman of the nineteenth century, Louis Pasteur and Antoine Béchamp.

A major area of difference between the drug approach to health care and the natural remedies approach is the way these two men viewed the activities of micro-organisms and their impact on health. In the middle of the nineteenth century Louis Pasteur identified and publicised infor-mation about the presence of bacteria and other pathogens at the site of infections. He then made the mental leap required to claim that the pathogen had caused the infection. Antoine Béchamp, also French and of a similar age, observed the same phenomenon but took the reverse view. He considered it was the breakdown of the terrain, the person's weakened or previously damaged tissues, that caused the disease and that the pathogens arrived later and were opportunistic beneficiaries rather than causative agents. Béchamp stated that this explained why one person succumbed to a particular health problem while another, in the same location or situation, did not.

The two men had many debates during the course of their profes-sional lives, but it is Pasteur who, at the end of his life, changed his mind and acknowledged 'It's the terrain that is important'.

Unfortunately, the initial ideas of Pasteur were seized upon by the many drug companies of the day and this continues to the present. It is easy to focus on finding drugs that are patentable and profitable and that will kill specific bugs or bacteria. Whether or not that ensures long-term health is debatable. On the other hand, it is impossible to make and patent profitable ways of improving the individual's terrain, for this depends on good diet, a healthy lifestyle and, if necessary, the use of nutrients, herbs and specific phytonutrient-rich foods, none of which can be patented. Thus the ideas of Béchamp were largely ignored, even though, in the end, Pasteur came round to them and embraced them.

Your health is linked to your terrain

CAM therapists follow the hypothesis put forward by Béchamp and, whatever your health problem, they work to improve the terrain: your body. This is why CAM therapists work with the whole body rather than focusing on a specific symptom or target tissue. It is also one of the reasons why CAM therapists put so much emphasis on diet, digestion, the avoidance of nutrient deficiencies and the removal of toxins, factors that are enormously important if you are to recover from cancer.

CAM, MDS or a Combination of the Two?

This is essentially a book about prevention and as such relates clearly to the CAM field. Therefore, there is little need to consider the ways in which the two systems can be combined. However, there is also the question of preventing recurrences, and if this is your concern it means you have had cancer and you may already have thought through the ideas concerning the possibility of combining the two therapeutic approaches; you may also still be on some form of MDS therapy. So, just for a moment, we will consider the arguments for one system or the other, or a combination of the two, in relation to the treatment of cancer. There is also the fact that if a person has received any of the MDS treatments this can also be considered a predisposing factor to a recurrence because:

1 After surgery there has to be tissue repair. This involves building new blood vessels (angiogenesis) to supply the new replacement tissue. However, the post-surgical angiogenic burst (when new blood vessels are rapidly made) can be excessive, and this may also increase the amount of capillary feed (blood and nutrients) to any remaining cancer cells.

2 Chemotherapy agents are strong cellular killers. In general they reduce immune function and damage the cells of the digestive tract and other rapidly dividing tissues. Some chemotherapy drugs can also cause cancer.[9]

3 Radiation is a known risk factor for cancer; for example, in one study of 31 women who had radiation for breast cancer, 19 (61 per cent) developed lung cancer, mostly on the same side, within 17 years.[10] Radiation treatment for Hodgkin's disease has been found to increase the subsequent risk of breast cancer.[11]

With two polar opposites to choose from, when you come to making decisions regarding your own health care, you cannot refuse to make a choice, for to refuse to choose is in itself to make a choice. It has to be you who makes the ultimate decision, no matter how much advice you take, for it is up to you whether or not you take that advice. Nor should you delegate that option, for it is you and your body that will be affected by the outcome, nobody else's. It is up to you whether your main focus is on drug medicine or the natural therapies, on the MDS system or the CAM therapies. You can, of course, combine the two, and this is often successful but, as you will learn, this is not always possible, and there are several ways where they can be seen to be working against each other.

Making the decision

To help you make your choice, it is useful to compare and contrast the differences. The following description is simplified and many people will be able to argue with some of the finer details, but in general the differences are as outlined below, with particular reference to cancer.

Attribute	Medical-drug-surgery (MDS) treatments	Complementary, alternative and metabolic (CAM) therapies
Focus on the specific symptoms	The tumour is usually the total focus	Although attention is paid to the tumour, the emphasis is on total body health. Your therapist will be looking for systemic and fundamental errors that need to be corrected.

Attribute	Medical-drug-surgery (MDS) treatments	Complementary, alternative and metabolic (CAM) therapies
Named diseases	A name given to a group of symptoms, often simply the Latin description, as in 'arthritis' for 'inflamed bones' or 'myasthenia gravis' for 'grave muscle' disease. This is not always helpful and may mask symptoms that are specific to the individual	CAM practitioners treat the whole person, and so are less interested in the name given to a specific group of symptoms
Consultation time	Most people report on feeling rushed, during the 7 or 9 minutes often allowed for a consultation	Consultations generally range from 30 minutes to an hour or more, so there is time for a whole-body approach and for full explanations
Focus on the whole body, not just the localised symptoms	Rarely, often made worse by time constraints, as well as by training omissions	Yes, an essential component of the CAM approach
Acute or emergency situations	Clearly your best option	CAM therapies come into play after the crisis is over, to aid recovery and prevent recurrence
Surgery	Excellent, when needed, and if a tumour is space-occupying and leading to collateral damage, but often overused. Biopsies and surgery can increase the risk of metastasis (secondary cancer growths). Surgery can induce excessive angiogenesis	Can often be avoided by the fundamental correction of the cause of the problem. There are other ways of reducing a tumour. If surgery is used, CAM supportive treatments can often hasten recovery
Pathogens (toxic organisms)	Considers that they are causative and should be destroyed, then all will be well	Considers the focus should be on why the body succumbed to the pathogens, and repairing that aspect, rather than simply killing the pathogens

Attribute	Medical-drug-surgery (MDS) treatments	Complementary, alternative and metabolic (CAM) therapies
Toxins	Unless there is a case of obvious and direct poisoning the MDS system pays little attention to toxins	Many toxic elements and compounds can interfere with the enzymes needed for normal cell function. Even low levels can be highly significant. The CAM therapist will try to identify any toxins and institute an appropriate detox programme to eliminate them. This is vital when you are endeavouring to break down tumours and destroy cancer cells
Prevention	Negligible understanding or emphasis. MDS practitioners have little to offer in this regard	A major component of the CAM approach. This applies to primary prevention and (secondary) prevention of a recurrence
Nutrition training	Essentially little or no nutrition components in their training	Nutrition and nutritional biochemistry are the foundation of most CAM therapies and occupy a significant proportion of the training
Diet and lifestyle teaching	Minimal and often incorrect	A major and essential part of treatment and education
Diet as part of therapy	Generally thought to be irrelevant	A vital part of the restoration of health
Treatments	Chemical drugs to act directly on a symptom	Nutrients, natural remedies and dietary components to restore total healthy functioning
Side effects	There is no MDS drug that does not have toxic side effects. Some are mild, others can be severe and even life-threatening	Almost all the side effects of CAM treatments are positive and provide additional benefits. Only in very rare situations of huge overdose are there even mild adverse side effects.
The mind–body connection	Generally ignored except for a recognition of the placebo effect	An integral part of most, or the best, CAM approaches

Attribute	Medical-drug-surgery (MDS) treatments	Complementary, alternative and metabolic (CAM) therapies
Psychotherapy	Generally none unless there are grounds for referral for a psychiatric condition	Stress lies behind a large proportion of cancers, and good CAM therapy always explores these avenues and encourages resolution of all stressful situations
Cost	High but usually hidden as it is generally paid for by either public or private insurance schemes	Generally born directly by the patient and so is more apparent. Usually significantly less than MDS treatments
Client involvement	Negligible. Many people report feeling disempowered by the process	Essential and encouraged. Harnessing the patient's involvement and understanding improves the outcome
Lifestyle changes	Negligible	Can be extensive depending on the nature of the original lifestyle
Long-term benefits or treatment	Variable, depending on the nature of the problem	Can be extensive, as the aim is fundamental emotional and lifestyle improvement and prevention of future problems

A combination

Except in very rare and unusual circumstances there is no reason why you should not combine all the concepts of Phase One of the cancer process with whatever MDS therapies you may choose to follow if you do have cancer. You can only improve your chances if you detect, attend to and remove all the predisposing factors.

There are other positive benefits of adding the CAM protocols to the MDS therapies. For instance, the use of curcumin in combination with radiation, in some situations, has been shown to improve the effectiveness of the radiation treatment[12] and reduce the incidence of radiation burns.

You may be told by your doctor or oncologist that antioxidants should not be used during chemotherapy. This is rarely based on solid evidence and is often a knee-jerk reaction against something outside their sphere of knowledge. If this is said to you, ask for the evidence or references that support the statements. The reason most commonly given is that many of the drugs used are strong oxidising agents and create their perceived benefit by creating toxic oxidising radicals within the cells, which includes, of course, healthy cells as well as cancer cells. This oxidising action would seem to be countered by nutrient antioxidants. There are two reasons why this is thought to be unlikely. Firstly, the oxidising effect of the chemotherapy agent is generally so strong that any effect of the plant antioxidants, in reducing the effect of the chemotherapy, would be negligible. What the antioxidants do achieve is to protect the rest of your body from excessive production of toxic oxygen free radicals. Secondly, many of the plant nutrients or active ingredients have collectively been lumped together and called 'antioxidants', when in fact many of them are not antioxidants at all but exert their benefit by entirely different mechanisms. This can cloud the issue unnecessarily.

There may sometimes be situations when a specific phytonutrient (an active plant nutrient) should not be combined with a specific chemical drug, but these are rare and details vary as we learn more about drug actions. In a great many more combinations the effects are improved by the supplements.

The efficacy or not of any individual combination of chemical drug and nutritional supplement will depend on (a) the type of MDS treatment; (b) the specific chemotherapy agents; (c) the specific nutritional supplement; (d) the type of cancer; (e) your own state of health, and more. This is a large subject and beyond the remit of this book. The information is continuously being upgraded by research, both into CAM therapies and into new chemotherapeutic agents, and so into their possible interactions. I would advise you to consult your CAM practitioner as to what would be best for you. In general, however, it is safe to say that most CAM therapies and treatments can usefully and beneficially be added to MDS treatments. Keep in mind, too, that many of the nutritional supplements you may want to take, such as vitamin D_3, vitamin C and essential minerals, as well as many of the active ingredients found in herbs and spices, such as turmeric, cayenne and garlic, are all found in food, and your oncologist will rarely tell you to stop eating such foods.

If you choose to have radiation treatments, by following the CAM approaches described here you can generally help to reduce some of the collateral damage that it causes.

Surgery

You might choose surgery, particularly if the tumour is large, but then decline to have either chemotherapy or radiation and turn, at that point, to CAM therapies. Surgery may be a sensible option, particularly in situations where a tumour is of such a size that it is interfering with other bodily functions. However, surgery is a major stress. By supporting the body with nutrients, plus healing and detox procedures, you can assist it through the process, help to reduce some of the damage that was inevitably caused and minimise any excessive angiogenic burst.

What about the disadvantages of combining the two approaches?

You may be heavily inclined towards the CAM approach and want to do all you can to make this successful, but at the same time you may feel safer if you also add in some aspects of the MDS system. If you want to take this option there are some factors to keep in mind.

In addition to the points already made, it is worth underlining the fact that the CAM approach is based on rebuilding and improving your immune system, whereas chemotherapy and radiation can have the reverse effect. The CAM approach is based on working with your body to build it up and improve it; the MDS treatments will damage your body.

With regard to tests, there is no essential conflict between the majority of the tests you will find discussed here and those your doctor may do. They are almost all laboratory tests, based on sound chemistry and physiology. However, although your CAM therapist will generally want all the information they can get and so will also be interested to know the results of all medical tests you have had done, as well as the tests they have organised themselves, your doctor will probably be less interested in the CAM tests, as they go beyond considerations of the tumour itself. There are, of course, some broad-thinking MDS professionals who, if they have had the training, can make very good use of the tests described here.

To recap

- If you are worried about developing cancer or about it recurring, the CAM approach can help you.
- Cancer is not only a tumour, it is a process, of which the tumour is the end result.
- There are two phases to this process: Phase One, comprised of predisposing factors that increase your risk of developing cancer; and Phase Two, in which cancerous cells are present and, usually, multiplying.
- The cancer process can be reversed.
- If you do have cancer, attacking the tumour is only part of the answer. It is essential that you also reverse the process that lead to its formation.
- CAM therapies and ideas can help you prevent the start of the process; they can also help you to reverse the process if it has started.

CHAPTER 5

Prevention — It's Critical

Are you doing all you can to look after your health? Or are you assuming that it is robust and will stand up to all you are currently throwing at it with your present diet and lifestyle? It is all too easy to take good health for granted when you have it, believing, at least subconsciously, that you will keep it forever.

For over 30 years I have been encouraging people to do all they can to prevent health problems. This means looking after and valuing the health that they have, and attending to the small details so that these do not develop into larger problems. It includes having regular check-ups and having the various tests that could warn of any impending problems. Yet more times than I can count I have heard people say, 'I'm healthy enough, there's nothing to worry about', or 'I'm healthy, I don't need check-ups.' Others say that they haven't the money, the time or, if the truth be told, the inclination, to bother with check-ups and prevention. Then they come back months or years later with problems, including cancer, that could have been prevented. In relation to cancer, people are less likely to want to find out about it than about many other potential health problems. Many people are too afraid to ask the question, because they are terrified of the answer. This is sad, because so many lives could be saved if people followed the suggestions for the tests and corrections that I will be describing in the following chapters.

Why You Need to Know

How do you know you are fully healthy at the cellular level without doing check-ups and without testing for the Vital Signs that can warn you of possible trouble? How do you know what subterranean rumblings there may be that have not yet caused an eruption on the surface?

As I write this, I have just learned of a woman who felt totally healthy five and a half weeks ago and who has now been diagnosed with several inoperable liver tumours, which are secondaries (metastatic) from an unknown primary tumour. Had she done, a year or more ago, some of the tests we will be covering here, she might have discovered the problem with sufficient time to turn it around.

In some ways the human body is tough and has amazing powers of both tolerance and recovery. This has many benefits, but it also has a major disadvantage. It means that you may have a number of problems developing and yet have no, or few, obvious symptoms to warn you of this. This can leave you in a fool's paradise, happily assuming that all is well when in fact there could be trouble brewing.

You maintain your car, but do you maintain your body? Imagine the scenario. You have won or been given a fabulous new car. You know you'd never be able to afford to purchase such a wonderful car for yourself and you're unlikely ever to have one again. You want this one to last as long as possible. What do you do? How do you care for it?

Do you fill it with inferior petrol, simply because it is cheaper, easier or quicker than buying the best? Do you wait to give it oil or water until the oil light has been on for a while and the engine is making strange sounds loudly enough that it bothers you to the point where you feel you had better do something about it, just to keep it quiet? Do you keep driving until there is an obvious problem? If there is one, do you think, *well, the performance hasn't gone down too much, the noise isn't too bad, I can live with it?* Do you wait until the problem is obviously serious, or until the car will no longer run?

I doubt it. Yet in effect that is what you do to your body when you fail to give it regular check-ups. With your body you wait until there are major symptoms of sufficient magnitude that you feel forced to see someone about them. All too often I hear patients saying such things as, 'I get a bit of indigestion, it's not too bad though, not worth worrying about', or 'I get a few headaches, but a few painkillers usually stops [suppresses] them and I can manage', or 'I have a pain in my chest, but it's not too bad . . . I'm sure it's nothing, not worth bothering a doctor about.' They forget that it's the doctor's job to be bothered. What causes the indigestion, the headache, the chest pain? If they had received regular check-ups these problems might not have started. If they have them checked the moment they start, the problems could be halted rather than allowed to develop further. Prevention is all important; it is infinitely easier to stop a problem at or near the start than to treat it once it has become serious.

Just as your car needs good-quality and clean oil, petrol and water to run well, so your body needs a good diet to run well and stay healthy. Most people look after their car better than they look after their health – and their car is replaceable; it can be traded in for a newer, younger model – their body cannot.

Your Diet Really is Important

There is an intimate connection between food and health. This is made clear in relation to cancer in that we know that at least 30 per cent of cancers are thought to be associated simply with a poor diet and with dietary problems.[13] It is amazing and illogical that, in spite of this, there is little or no emphasis by the MDS profession on using dietary improvements as a part of their treatment protocols.

Roland S	During a discussion with Roland and his wife on what diet would best help them while he was having chemotherapy, I warned that 'sugar feeds cancer' and that he should avoid it entirely. (This is explained in Chapter 17.) They later asked the nurse in the hospital about it, but all she could say was 'I don't know of any reason why he can't eat sugar; we all eat it, it can't do him any harm.' How wrong she was. Fortunately the patient realised this.

I have yet to find a client who eats a truly, 100 per cent, good diet. Some eat dreadful diets, some eat poor diets and some eat good diets part of the time and then let their standards drop at others. As one client typically put it, 'I eat well all week, so I figure it doesn't matter if I don't bother at weekends when I'm out socialising and having a good time.' My response was simple, 'You do freelance work don't you? How would you feel if every fifth contractor didn't pay you, saying that as the other four had done so you could manage without his fee?' She was, of course, aghast at the idea – but got the point.

Do you do some of the positive things (diet or supplements) some of the time but not all of them all of the time? I have a friend and colleague who (generally but not always) eats fairly well and who (most of the time) takes supplements. When I once commented that I was surprised that she ate white bread rolls, bars of chocolate and sweet custard tarts in between her good meals she replied that as she took supplements it wouldn't matter if she ate badly from time to time. This, too, is to miss the point entirely. You wouldn't put top-quality petrol in your car some of the time and then feel that meant it was acceptable to put cheap or poor-quality petrol in at other times just because it had some extra additives in it.

Adding Extra: Supplements

You might put additives into your petrol to ensure the smooth running of the engine. But do you think about the additives or supplements you need for your body? Perhaps you never take them, or perhaps you take them occasionally and sporadically, and without a lot of attention to detail. Are you taking the ones that you need? Are you taking some that you don't need, which could unbalance the others? The tests we will be discussing in the coming chapters will help you to decide which supplements you need.

Many of my clients have explained that they were taking the cheapest supplements to save money. Would you do that to your car? Almost certainly not. Ironically, the supplements that are apparently the cheapest generally work out to be the most costly. Here's why. The fixed costs of getting the capsules into their bottles, into the shops and marketing them are the same, whatever the cost of the ingredients. If you double or treble the cost of the ingredients, the cost of the final product will not increase in the same way; it may only go up by around 10 or 20 per cent. In the end, the better quality and stronger product is generally the most economical.

Why Regular 'Servicing' is Best

What about the costs of regular servicing? Although health tests may cost you money, getting sick will cost even more, both directly and indirectly. The aim of this book is to alert you to the numerous ways in which you can run maintenance checks on yourself. The tests recommended here will tell you about early warning signs and problems long before they manifest as a full-blown disease or tumour. The results obtained from these tests, by their very nature, will point you in the right direction for fundamental correction. This will give you time to turn back from the direction in which you are heading before you get seriously ill.

Katie R | Katie had decided early on in life to stick to a good diet, take a supplement programme, take steady exercise and do whatever she could to maintain her health. She therefore insisted she was healthy and didn't need to do any tests, in spite of minor digestive problems. A year after her first visit she returned having had a spate of slightly worse digestive problems, which she still insisted were not much – a bit of an upset stomach, slightly constipated, lacking in energy. All she wanted was some digestive enzymes or some herbs to take for her problems. This time I was able to persuade her to do some tests; she agreed, although somewhat reluctantly. A stool analysis showed up a number of problems, the worst of which was the presence of blood. This, on investigation, turned out to be due to a tumour in the colon. Only then did she wish she had done the earlier testing for, as she now realises, the lack of symptoms or the presence of only minor ones, does not necessarily mean that everything is perfect.

Many people bury their head in the sand with regard to their own health. It is easier to take the it-won't-happen-to-me attitude and continue to follow what is regarded as a normal lifestyle, until 'happen' is just what it does. However, there is a positive side to the testing, because all the prevention strategies lead not just to a reduced risk of developing cancer but also to better overall health.

CAM therapies have side effects, but, unlike those of drugs, the side effects are all good. When you pay proper attention to your health, and detect and sort out any underlying problems, you may be amazed at how much better you can feel. Clients come back after treatment saying that they have more energy, their digestion has settled down, their skin has improved, their mood is better, they have better memory and concentration and they are more motivated to do things. They may even tell me of the resolution of problems they had failed to mention to me at the start.

Tina S

> Tina did all that was indicated by the tests she undertook for abdominal pain, and then found that her straight, grey hair had regained some of its original brown tones and curl, and that her astigmatism was corrected.

Keeping it Going

Finally, there is maintenance. You may have found a problem and then corrected it, but what do you do next? I frequently work with patients who have come to my office with a health problem, and who start on a healthy regime and feel very much better. I'm then asked, 'How long will I have to follow this programme?' This is MDS-think: have symptom – take drug to eliminate symptom – revert to old lifestyle – expect to stay well. It makes no sense. My answer to the question is generally, 'For as long as you want to feel well rather than ill and to be healthy rather than to revert to your previous deteriorating health.'

Where Are You Now?

You may feel that you *should* be healthy because your current diet and lifestyle are 'normal'. Because you know that 'everyone else does it', you may think that what you are currently doing is therefore acceptable. However 'normal' it seems, though, think about your diet. Is it full of highly processed foods with lots of fats and refined carbohydrates such as white flour, white rice and sugars? Do you rarely eat vegetables and fruits? Do you often eat fast foods, or eat 'on the run'? And what about the other harmful things that you can do to your body – alcohol, caffeine, tobacco and more – how often do you have these?

Look at your lifestyle as well. In our modern lives it is indeed 'normal' for most of us to spend hours on our mobile phones, to live enmeshed in a pulsing electro-magnetic field of computers and electrical equipment, to breathe polluted air, bombard our bodies with a range of medical drugs, and slather our skins with chemically laden toiletries and cosmetics (see box opposite). Many of us live a sedentary life. These things are common, and they may be the norm, but they are not normal or healthy.

A word about 'chemical'

You will often hear or read the word 'chemical' used pejoratively, as above. Our world, including our bodies and all our foods, is made up of chemicals. Some are essential, some are beneficial and some are harmful. By common usage, in this context, such terms as 'chemical' and 'chemicals' in relation to foods, cosmetics, cleaners, and so on, have come to mean substances that are actually or potentially toxic or carcinogenic, certainly substances that are foreign to the body and potentially harmful.

Remember that cancer cells will not be detected by the MDS system until there are a billion or more of them, and only then if you are having a high-tech scan such as an MRI or a PET or CAT scan. There may have to be billions of billions of these cells before you have a tumour that can lead to symptoms that will send you to your practitioner. So what can you do? Detect the Vital Signs, do the tests described in the following pages, and act on the results.

Cancer is common. The number of people killed in the UK by cancer each year (155,488 in 2007,[14]) is equivalent to more than the full complement of a Jumbo 747 (approximately 400 passengers) crashing every day with a total loss of life, or to one 9/11 World Trade Center event happening every week. Imagine the headlines that would make.

You are at a higher risk of getting cancer than of almost any other health problem. Learning how to prevent it by identifying any of the predisposing factors of Phase One is a major step in the prevention of the fully cancerous activity of Phase Two.

Making Changes

Early detection is critical. You can be comforted by the fact that there is a huge body of peer-review, evidence-based research, that clearly demonstrates that you can have a significant impact on the predisposing factors and that you can hope either to turn the cancer process around or halt its progress, certainly before it has reached the tumour stage. There is even a very real chance that you can turn it around once it has reached the tumour stage, but this is generally accomplished with greater difficulty.

Cancer, if you do get it, can generally be managed, rather like diabetes, if you are willing to do what it takes. But it takes a lot. Much may be demanded of you to first overcome it and then to stay in remission, in time, energy, lifestyle disciplines and money. It is far better to prevent it from starting.

Some practitioners, in both systems, but particularly in the CAM system, recognise that the term 'cure' may be unrealistic when applied to cancer once it has occurred. They acknowledge that there may always be some cancer cells present in an affected individual, but that they can be kept under control by all the methods discussed here aimed at both pre-vention (primary and of a recurrence) and at improving your general health. This may mean you have to implement several long-term lifestyle changes and an ongoing programme of detox, diet and supplements. These may not 'cure' the condition entirely, any more than diabetes is cured when it is managed by insulin or other drugs, yet they may halt its progress and mean you can continue to live a full and active life, if careful, well into old age. You may well even be healthier than you would otherwise have been, as a result of all the strategies and lifestyle changes you put in place.

———————————

It's time now to consider the early warning signs, the predisposing fac-tors, that could be leading you, at least potentially, in the direction of degenerative diseases in general and of cancer in particular.

PART 2
WHAT TO DO AND HOW MUCH AT RISK ARE YOU?

CHAPTER 6

Your Anti-Cancer Programme

In this chapter I give you a quick overview of the chapters to come. As you read through the steps below you may find one or more that you feel are particularly relevant to yourself or to someone about whom you are concerned. If this is the case you can jump ahead to the appropriate chapter.

Before You Start

Check that you have not moved into Phase Two of the cancer process. In the next chapter (Chapter 7) you will learn of a test, called CA Profile, that will tell you whether or not you have moved from Phase One – the precancerous phase that applies to everyone who has not developed cancer – and into Phase Two. The CA Profile is an invaluable test and, if used as a monitoring tool and the results acted upon, could save many lives.

Even if the results of this CA Profile are normal, you need to apply all that is discussed in the following chapters. Just as I am recommending that you do not wait for a tumour to form before you become concerned about having cancer, I also recommend that you do all you can to prevent the development of even the earliest precancerous cells that can be detected by the CA Profile. In addition, correcting any of the predisposing factors that apply to you will help you to avoid many other health problems, as they are all aimed at improving your overall general health.

Your strategies for achieving optimum health will vary depending on your starting position.

Step 1: Improve Your Diet

It is almost certain that your diet is not perfect, so this is the time to improve the situation. In Chapters 9 and 10 you will learn how to determine your metabolic type, so that you can find which are the best foods for you, as an individual, to eat. The main dietary instructions are given in a table on pages 77–81 but the key points are:

1   Cut out all forms of sugar and refined carbohydrates (such as white flour and white rice, and their products).

2   Cut out processed vegetable oils, such as sunflower or corn oil, and overheated fats, such as those that have been heated to smoking temperature or used for deep-fat frying, or fats that have been 'burned to a crisp'. Choose coconut oil, flaxseed and olive oil instead.

3   Eat only organic foods. If you cannot do this, at least avoid processed foods that contain chemical additives.

4   Make vegetables the main part of your diet and eat much of your diet in the form of raw food to preserve the valuable enzymes and other nutrients.

Step 2: Correct Any Nutrient Deficiencies

Even the best food you can find cannot provide you with all the nutrients you need for optimum health. This is discussed in Chapters 11 and 12. Do the ONE test, as described in Chapter 10 and correct any vitamin and mineral deficiencies that are indicated.

Step 3: Improve Your Digestion

It is one thing to swallow all the foods and nutrients you need, but this is of little use if you do not properly digest the foods and absorb the nutrients. In Chapter 13 you will learn more about the way your digestive system functions, what can go wrong, how to detect any errors and how to correct them. By these means you can prevent a number of more serious problems that could otherwise develop.

Step 4: Support Your Liver

Your liver has more jobs to do than any other organ in your body. It is an essential part of your digestive system, and it is the absolute core of your ability to eliminate toxins. It bears the brunt of many of your bad habits, including excessive alcohol consumption, eating processed and heated fats and being overburdened by all the toxins you take in. If you know you have been giving your liver a hard time, then ease up on it. It is a forgiving organ and can often recover from some of the challenges you throw at it, but it can't do this indefinitely. This is fully discussed in Chapter 14.

Step 5: Get Rid of Toxins

In the modern world it is impossible to avoid toxins. In the cities there are industrial and domestic pollutants. In the countryside there are agricultural and wind-borne pollutants. The best you can do is to avoid what you can and then include some detoxing processes into your regular routine so that your body can eliminate the toxins that you cannot avoid. In Chapter 15 you will find a discussion of some of the toxins to which you may be exposed, details of the tests you can do to determine the toxins already present in your body, and a number of procedures to help you eliminate them. Briefly, here are the recommendations covered:

1   Go on a comprehensive detox programme. You will inevitably choose your own detox methods and many different ones are given in Chapter 15.

2   If you are seriously concerned about toxins, then do the various tests indicated for them so that you know exactly what you have to deal with.

3   Enemas may seem unnatural, but then so is much of the modern lifestyle. An occasional or even a daily enema, depending on your state of health, can help to reduce your toxic load. This is becoming an increasingly common practice among people concerned about cancer.

4   Select the other detox suggestions that appeal to you and that you can work into your daily routine.

Step 6: Correct Your Energy Production and Your Sugar Metabolism

Cancer seriously disrupts your energy production, and this topic is discussed in Chapter 16. Once you understand this mechanism, and the way that cancer cells use glucose (discussed in Chapter 17), you will better understand why you should absolutely eliminate all sugars from your diet.

Step 7: Balance Your Neurotransmitters, Reduce Your Stress Levels and Give Your Adrenal Glands a Chance

We now know that your brain 'speaks' chemically to almost all the cells in your body. In Chapter 18 you will learn about neurotransmitters, the messenger chemicals that travel from your brain to the cells of the various and different parts of your body. It is generally recognised that many cancers become apparent two or three years after periods of extreme stress (see Chapter 19). So, learn to relax, to meditate, to take time out and to have fun – and how to make your heart sing. Exhausted adrenal glands are a prime cause of several problems that generate triggers which convert healthy cells into cancer cells. This is the subject of Chapter 20.

Step 8: Correct Any Other Predisposing Factors

There are, of course, many other predisposing factors. The main ones of these include an underactive thyroid gland (Chapter 21), an under-functioning immune system (Chapter 22) and faulty oestrogen metabolism (Chapter 23).

Step 9: Reduce Your Risk Factors

Risk factors differ from predisposing factors. They are those activities, situations or other triggers that increase your likelihood of developing cancer. They are generally recognised as such. Cigarette smoking, a lack of exercise and being overweight are obvious examples (see Chapter 8). Some of the risk factors, such as age, sex and past events in your life you cannot change, but I urge you to change the ones that you can. If you don't make these changes, you may later wish you had.

If you think you need help, find a practitioner who understands the cancer process. When you have done all this and organised your new lifestyle, sit back, relax, and have fun. Remember, filling your life with joy and pleasure is an important aspect of preventing cancer.

A. To improve your chances of avoiding cancer:

Follow through the discussion of Phase One, and do as many tests as you feel inclined to do or that seem appropriate to your present state of health. Make all the appropriate changes and adjustments to your diet and lifestyle as are needed, based on your results. If necessary, correct any of the predisposing factors that may be present.

If you are concerned that you may have already developed cancer, do the CA Profile test described in Chapter 7. This panel, and particularly its component tests for compounds called HCG and PHI (discussed more fully later) is possibly the best early warning generalised set of tests we have for cancer, anywhere in the body. If that test is clear, you can generally relax, but you should, of course, maintain the improvements in your lifestyle that you have introduced. They are an ongoing part of prevention.

B. If you have had cancer and are in remission:

Firstly, you should follow A above. Cancer is not like measles; having it once does not mean that you have developed immunity to it. If you are in remission, a recurrence is still possible. Even if you are totally clear of your first cancer, your risk of getting cancer in the future is the same as it is for anyone who hasn't had cancer: around 40 per cent, depending on the statistics you read.

If, as a result of having had cancer, you have already taken steps to improve your health and lifestyle, you may have improved your odds, but against this is the fact that you have shown that your body was quite capable of developing cancer once and may, for similar reasons, readily develop it again if the triggers are there. So, follow through on all the ideas relating to Phase One. Do the CA Profile. If the results of this test are abnormal, even if you have no detectable tumour, and even if your doctors and oncologists say you are in full remission, you are not in the clear. All the evidence that we have indicates that you still have some cancer cells and you should work towards complete remission at the cellular (microscopic) level.

C. If you have cancer:

Work with all the chapters in this book. Cancer is an ongoing process. All the time you have it, new cancer cells are constantly forming. Your immediate task is to prevent this happening, to slow down, then stop and hopefully reverse the process. Eliminating the predisposing factors will rebuild your overall health so that all the other strategies have a much better chance of success.

It is also very important that you find a practitioner to work with. If the ideas discussed here make sense to you, you will want to find a practitioner that understands these concepts and knows how to apply them. Although the following pages will give you a lot of information that you can use yourself, cancer is much too serious a problem for you to deal with on your own. This is clearly true if you know little or nothing about CAM health care, it is also true if you already feel that you know a lot. It is even true if you are a practitioner, for no matter how well qualified you are, there is more out there that you can learn, and you also need a different perspective. It is difficult for anyone to be objective about themselves.

In addition to whatever treatment programme you choose to adopt, you should do the various tests described or listed here for Phase One; all these tests can be used to monitor the progress you are making. Even once the test results are all back to normal, including your results of the CA Profile, you should continue with whatever positive steps you have been taking, to maintain these achievements.

Take supplements daily

Eating 'cures' hunger but you do not expect to be able to stop eating, long term, once your hunger is appeased; you have an ongoing daily need for food. It is the same with supplements. As their name implies, they are a supplement to your daily diet. You take them, get an improvement, but then have to recognise that this improvement is based on the fact that you are taking them. Just as you have to eat every day, if you want to maintain good health you have to continue daily with the supplements and the other good habits that have helped you to improve your health.

That, in brief, is an indication of the steps we will be exploring as we work through Part Three. First, however, it is pertinent to consider what tests you can do to detect the possibility of cancer having started, before there is any tumour large enough to be detected.

CHAPTER 7

Do You Have Cancer?

Having come this far you may well be wondering whether or not you have already started along the cancer process. You assuredly have progressed along Phase One, as already explained. We all have. It is merely a question of how far. The bigger question is whether or not you have moved from Phase One to Phase Two.

You will probably know already of some of the tests you can do to check that you don't have specific types of cancer. Mammograms can detect early breast tumours. A PAP smear (also known as the papanicola test) can warn of impending cervical cancer. A test for raised PSA (prostate specific antigen) can warn of prostate problems. There are also tumour markers that can be detected in a blood test, such as CA125 for ovarian cancer or CA 15-3 for breast cancer, and so on.

These tests are more or less specific to individual types of cancer. However, they can also be present when the tumour is somewhere other than its usual source. For instance the presence of CEA (cancer embryonic antigen) most commonly suggests a cancer within the digestive tract, usually the colon, but it can also be found occasionally when there is a tumour in the lungs or breast.

These tests may indicate the presence and probable location of a tumour. This is helpful if the main thrust of any treatment you may choose will be to attack or remove the tumour. However, the thesis of this book is that you should be looking for any earlier warning signs, signs that alert you to the possibility that Phase Two of the cancer process has started, whether or not there is a significant or detectable tumour yet present. If you are focusing on the process that could be leading to a tumour, to the early stages of the cancer process, there are several drawbacks to relying on these tumour markers as your early-warning signs:

- They do not tell you about the very early changes at the cellular level in general.
- They only tell you about, dominantly, one type of cancer.

- To get a full coverage you would have to test for tumour markers for all the tissues in which a tumour could develop. That presents two problems: (a) the markers don't all exist; and (b) the cost would be prohibitive, even for doing them all once, but certainly for frequent monitoring or prevention.

Fortunately, there are some tests that can give you a more general picture of the possibility that some of your cells are starting to turn cancerous. The CA Profile, already mentioned and discussed below, is an example, and although it is not the only test available it is the one that, at the time of writing, has given the best early warning sign of cancer in general for an economical price. A new cancer test that takes 30 minutes and uses a special chip was reported on in *Nature Nanotechnology* in October 2009;[15] however, this is still in the research and development phase. Research is ongoing and you would be wise to look out for further developments in this area. In the meantime, thousands of people have done the CA Profile and the results have been extremely useful.

The CA Profile

The CA Profile© is offered by American Metabolic Laboratories (see Resources). Its main component is a set of three tests, two using a blood (serum only) and one using a urine sample, for different forms of a hormone called human chorionic gonadotropin or HCG. This is well accepted in medical circles as an indicator of one type of cancer, of choriocarcinoma, or the cancer that can occur in pregnancy if excessive early embryonic growth is not stopped and this pregnancy-related cancer occurs.

Dr John Beard, an English embryologist, as far back as 1905, postulated that placental tissue is the same as cancerous tissue and so laid the groundwork for the recognition that HCG, associated with placental tissue, is also associated with all types of cancer. Although this was generally denied within the MDS system throughout the twentieth century, a growing number of oncologists are now beginning to accept this.

HCG is the hormone that is tested for in the common pregnancy test, but if you are pregnant, your level of this hormone will be very much higher than if you have cancer. For this reason the pregnancy testing kit need not be as sensitive as the test for cancer and so it is of no use for you in this context.

HCG is a complex molecule made up of more than one sub-unit. Although other laboratories may do the test, if it is not designed specifically to detect the cancer aspects of this hormone it will not give you reliable results. This is where the long history of research and development of American Metabolics is useful. The laboratory is located in America, but it is easy to send the samples there, and they provide full instructions as to how this should be done. You will need a practitioner, either CAM or medical, to authorise the test, but they can readily arrange this by contacting the laboratory for you.

American Metabolics has undertaken extensive research and has developed a procedure that will detect the very small amounts of HCG. They say:

> HCG can be elevated in an existing cancer, stress that is leading to cancer, or in a developing cancer, in some instances as many as ten to twelve years before an actual tumour could be detected by any other method. Normal levels are less than 1.0 mlU/mL. A grey zone, i.e. a less certain zone is between 1.0 and 3.0 mlU/mL. Results above 3.0 mlU/mL should be seriously considered. It is known that it may take ten to twelve years to develop cancer, so an HCG elevation may indicate that an individual may be anywhere in this time range.[16]

They go on to say that 'even though the CA Profile is the best of its kind, giving positive results in 90–93 per cent of established cancer cases, a pathologist does the final diagnosis on tissue/cell biopsy analysis.'

If your results are below 1.0 mlU/mL you can be reasonably sure that you do not have any permanent cancer cells and that you are not currently in Phase Two, although you would be wise to repeat the test every year or two to be sure your situation has not changed.

The HCG result is setting the scene. If it is high, it suggests that you are highly susceptible to developing cancer and that whenever a major trigger occurs, such as a significant stress, an illness that overloads your immune system or exposure to significant carcinogens, for example, then tumour development is likely and could accelerate. At worst, it suggests that you already have cancer.

Additional tests

This CA Profile includes other tests. One of these is for an enzyme called PHI (phosphohexose isomerase). This enzyme is active in the EM (Embden–Meyerhoff) pathway, which is explained in Chapter 16. You will learn there that this pathway is the anaerobic (oxygen-free) first phase of glucose breakdown that takes place in the cytosol of your cells, as opposed to the major pathway, the aerobic phase that takes place in the mitochondria. Cancer cells rely on, and so promote, the anaerobic phase, so an abnormal amount of PHI is indicative of activity that is characteristic of cancer cells rather than healthy cells. If there is an abnormal increase in the amount of PHI present it suggests that there is an excessive amount of anaerobic activity in your cells – activity that is characteristic of cancer cells rather than of healthy cells.

As stated by American Metabolics in their report that comes with the test results:

> PHI can be elevated in a developing cancer, existing cancer, or an acute heart, liver, muscle disease, acute hypothyroidism or acute viral infection. Examples of these acute conditions are myocardial infarction, hepatitis, AIDS, and traumatic muscle injury. If an acute condition can be ruled out, cancer may be the cause of the elevated result and the ten to twelve year cancer developmental clock may be ticking.[17] [Note the emphasis on acute rather than chronic conditions.]

CEA (cancer embryonic antigen) mentioned on page 54, is included in this panel of tests. GGTP (or gamma-glutamyltransferase) is an enzyme that is commonly used to assess liver function, although it may also be raised in diseases of the heart, lungs or kidneys. A raised level suggests possible liver damage, or reduced liver function; you will learn how important your liver is for your health in general and for removing toxins from your body in Chapters 14 and 15. An unhealthy liver is a predisposing factor for cancer.

DHEA is another compound that is included in the test. Your level of DHEA falls as your adrenal glands become progressively more and more stressed, and also with age. A low level, and especially a low level for your age, indicates the probability of adrenal exhaustion, and in Chapter 20 you will learn about the vital importance of having healthy adrenal glands and not being overly stressed. TSH or thyroid-stimulating hormone is the hormone that stimulates your thyroid gland into action. If its level is outside the normal range this will provide information as to your thyroid function, and in Chapter 21 you will discover how important this gland is. Poor function of either the adrenals or thyroid gland is a significant predisposing factor.

The group of tests as a whole package, although not cheap, is reasonably priced and it provides a useful first step if you want to check on the possibility that you might be in the earliest stages of Phase Two of the cancer process.

The AMAS Test

You may have read about the AMAS (anti-malignin antibody) test. It measures the level of an antibody (a protein produced by your immune system) in the blood, called anti-malignin. It was found that the level of this antibody was high in some people with cancer and it was hoped that the presence of these antibodies would constitute an early warning sign for the start of the development of cancer cells; however, the results have been ambiguous and it is generally not considered safe to rely solely on this test as a test for the presence or absence of cancer. Present indications are that the CA Profile is a more useful and reliable test.

———————————

To summarise so far, we've looked at some of the basic information regarding the nature of cancer as seen from a CAM perspective. I've suggested that cancer is a process leading eventually to the end product of a final tumour. Finally, I've outlined a simple approach to determining whether or not you could already be in Phase Two of the cancer process. It is now time to focus on the main topic of this book, the predisposing factors that constitute Phase One and the tests you can do to help you eliminate them and increase your ability to prevent cancer.

PART 3
THE
PREDISPOSING
FACTORS

CHAPTER 8

Predisposing Factors and Risk Factors

As well as leading to cancer, predisposing factors can lead to the development of a variety of other degenerative diseases. Although none of them, on their own, need necessarily lead to cancer, your body can only withstand a limited number of such predisposing factors before the last straw, the final stress, carcinogen or genetic change, tips you over into Phase Two. It may take only one predisposing factor of sufficient magnitude, but this is rare. In general, a number of them will be operating. This is useful, as you can start to improve all of them at once, creating a cumulatively positive effect as the various aspects of your health improve and revert to optimum function.

When you drive down a cul-de-sac, the only sensible method of escape is to reverse back the way you have come. Forcing your car through bushes may get you to the other side, but only with serious damage to your car. You must reverse out, but that may not be enough. Reversing out does not repair the damage your car may have acquired on the way in or clean off the mud from unsuspected potholes, so cleaning and repairs may be needed. It is the same with your body. More fundamental corrections will have to be made. If a poor diet and nutritional deficiencies have led to symptoms of degeneration, then the way to reverse back into better health is to improve your diet, increase your nutrient intake and not to take toxic drugs. In addition, you will have to adopt other therapies to correct the collateral damage that has been done.

In the pages ahead you will find a range of tests that you can do, or ask for, to give you guidance on which parts of your body need attention, and you will find suggestions as to how to go about reversing into, and restoring, good health.

One of the problems with prevention is that it is nearly always impossible to know what you have prevented. So, you will find that many tests are recommended. By doing the tests that follow, both before and after your treatment or correctional interventions, you can know whether or not you have improved a system that was faulty and resolved a problem that was otherwise likely to get worse.

Although an enormous number of tests could be done, I base my emphasis here on the following criteria:

- The tests are readily available and accessible.
- The tests can warn you of impending problems.
- You can act, based on the results. You can do something positive to correct any errors that are found, and in general these remedies lie within the CAM field.

Risk Factors Versus Predisposing Factors

We all know about risk factors. These are the various lifestyle and genetic factors that, if present, increase your risk of developing cancer. There is a difference between predisposing factors and risk factors. Risk factors are self-evident. In general, once you are told about them you can readily recognise whether or not they relate to you. You do not need tests to do this. Here are just a few examples.

The risk factors that you can change

Firstly, the ones that you do have some control over:

Alcohol consumption – in excess

Arguably all alcohol applies a stress to the liver and is toxic. Equally there are suggestions that drinking either one or two, but no more, 175 ml glasses of red wine a day may not do significant harm and may even do some good. It helps you to relax, improves social situations, applies the 'feel-good factor' and, specific to red wine, provides resveratrol, a beneficial bioflavonoid that helps prevent all three stages of cancer development: initiation, promotion and progression.[18]

Cigarette smoking

There is now a clear link between cigarette smoking and not only lung cancer but also a number of other cancers.

Lack of exercise

A sedentary lifestyle is a risk factor. Even half an hour's walking a day can reduce your risk of developing cancer. Do more if you can. For maximum benefit it should be aerobic exercise, such that your breathing rate increases but you do not become totally out of breath. The latter would indicate that you have moved over into anaerobic exercise and this is not helpful because cancer cells thrive in anaerobic conditions.

Hormone treatments

The use of hormone treatments – the oral contraceptive pill and HRT – are thought to increase your risk of cancer as well as some other degenerative diseases.[19]

Obesity

Being overweight is a serious predisposing factor for many types of cancer, including breast and prostate. Libraries of books have been written about weight and weight management, and if you are overweight you should consult these, obtain advice, join a club or do whatever it takes to get your weight down to normal.

These, and others, are risk factors. You know if they apply to you. So if you want to do your utmost to avoid cancer you should change these behaviours.

Risk factors you cannot change

You can't change your age or your sex. You can't change your history with regard to the number of babies you have had, the amount of breast feeding you have done, or the number of sexual partners you have had, yet all these can affect your risk of specific types of cancer. Having had your gall bladder out can be a risk factor for right-side colon cancer,[20] but this is not something you can change if you have already had the operation. However, knowledge of these risk factors may change decisions you make about actions in your future.

Predisposing factors

The predisposing factors are different to your risk factors in that they relate to your underlying health, to ongoing issues that can only be detected in adequate detail by doing the tests and by recognising the Vital Signs. You need tests to determine which diet is best for you, the existence of nutrient deficiencies, the presence of toxins, whether you have exhausted adrenal glands, an underactive thyroid gland or impending diabetes. It is the tests, described in this book, that constitute the Vital Signs of predisposing factors that can warn you of impending problems. Armed with this knowledge, and some of the treatment indications given here, you can improve your health in general.

In the chapters that follow I will explain the various predisposing factors.

CHAPTER 9

Predisposing Factor No. 1 – A Poor Diet

The quality of your food dictates, to a large measure, the structure and functional health of your body. This should be so obvious as to not need stating or stressing, yet it is almost invariably ignored by most of the medical profession.

So, the first factor predisposing you to cancer, as well as to all other health problems, is a bad diet. If your diet is bad you are almost certainly heading for a range of health problems. Positive dietary changes can be a lot more powerful than you might think.

Malcolm I

My very first patient with cancer, back in the early 1980s, was Malcolm, in his mid sixties. He had extensive lymphatic cancer when he first came to see me and his oncologist had given him five months to live. His cardiologist did not think he would live that long and predicted only four months. No treatment was deemed to be appropriate or worth attempting by his medical advisors. He had been treated by a wonderful Sydney-based Greek doctor, Dr Archie Kalokerinos, author of *Every Second Child*, a story of vitamin C and the improved survival of Aboriginal infants. Dr Kalokerinos had been giving Malcolm intravenous vitamin C (80g a week) plus oral vitamin C and a range of nutrients, but when he left Sydney he referred Malcolm to me.

Malcolm was an excellent potter, and prior to his diagnosis had just returned from Australia's Northern Territory with notes for his next book on Aboriginal artwork. He was saddened to think that he no longer had any energy and that the book would not be written.

We had far fewer tools then to deal directly with cancer than we have now. This, in effect, meant that what we could do was essentially to apply all the prevention techniques we had and remove all the predisposing factors that were present, and hope that that was sufficient. I changed his diet, radically, and added a more extensive range of nutrients, a range of herbal and homoeopathic remedies and suggested several detox techniques, but I could not, of course, give him intravenous vitamin C, because this is a medical prerogative. A year later, to our mutual delight, he was clear on all counts and he finished his book, a copy of which I still treasure.

He had a wonderfully positive attitude, which almost certainly helped. At one point he had decided to learn hydroponics and told me, 'I'm too busy with this gardening now to think about having cancer. Cancer will have to wait.'

A few years later he and his wife had moved into the Australian bush, 400 miles from Sydney, and he was back to potting with a foot wheel, and hewing wood in a way few people of his age could manage. When I was in the vicinity they insisted I visit for the day. I offered to help them get lunch – as one does in the Outback. 'What have you planned for lunch?' I asked.

'Salad – you told us to eat salad every day.'

'With what?'

'A small amount of meat – you told us to eat our protein for breakfast and lunch but not for dinner'

'What else do you want in the salad?'

'Alfalfa sprouts – you told us to eat them daily and they're over there, in the jars, the way you told us to grow them.'

'What oil do you use for the dressing?'

'Flaxseed oil – you told us to, and to keep it in the deep freeze.'

'Where is the flour you want for the sauce you plan?'

'In the "room temperature" fridge as you advised' (the outdoor temperature being nearer to 40°C (105°F) but a cold refrigerator being too cold).

It continued. Spending time with them was like seeing every single suggestion I had ever made to them, no matter how casually or how trivial, made manifest in their home. It was little wonder to me that he had returned to such good health. After 14 years his health did deteriorate and I heard from his family that he had died quite suddenly, probably due to his heart, aged nearly eighty.

He remains a testimony to the power of removing the predisposing factors.

Never underestimate the power of a good diet, especially if you are as meticulous as Malcolm was.

Is your diet good? Probably not. Is it perfect? Highly unlikely. Is it the right diet for you? Possibly, but it could almost certainly be made more appropriate.

The Metabolic-Type Diet

Eating the foods that are wrong for you is a predisposing factor. So, the first step is to determine just which foods suit your own unique metabolism. You may have come across books that offer to show you whether you are a protein or carbohydrate type. This is a start, but it is not enough. You may have come across others that talk about the blood-group diet. They tell you that if you are blood group O you should eat more meat, if you are blood group A you should tend towards a vegetable-based diet with fish. If you are blood group B you do well on dairy products, and if you are blood group AB you can eat a mixed diet. This can be helpful, but it is still too generalised.

Fortunately, there are better solutions and ones that can be tailored to you personally. For one of these go to www.healthexcel.com and follow the signs to determine your metabolic type. For a fee, you will have various screens of questions to answer, then you will be told via email which of the six main types you are. You will be given a table of foods with indications as to which ones are (a) terrific for you; (b) good for you; (c) all right as long as they are only eaten occasionally; and (d) to be totally avoided. Choose foods from the first two categories as much as possible.

There are six metabolic types, as defined by this questionnaire, but even within each type there are also subtle differences as to exactly which foods will be recommended for you. The types are called:

1   Parasympathetic dominants
2   Sympathetic dominants
3   Balanced autonomics
4   Fast oxidisers
5   Slow oxidisers
6   Mixed oxidatives

To understand what these terms mean you need to know a little about how your body functions.

The autonomic nervous system

If you are one of the first three types, your metabolism is controlled by your autonomic (think automatic) nervous system. This system, for our present purpose, can be divided into two distinct sections. One of these, your sympathetic nervous system (SNS) deals with the outside world: your fight or flight mechanism. It responds to challenges. Historically, such stresses or challenges meant either running away or giving chase, usually accompanied by some other sort of physical activity, including fighting. When this system is triggered, blood is sent to your limbs (to run and fight) to your eyes (for better acuity) and to your lungs (to increase oxygen uptake and availability). This blood has to come from somewhere, and the obvious place is your abdomen.

While you are dealing with this external challenge you do not want to be wasting energy digesting food or preparing urine. You certainly do not have time to stop and eliminate wastes. Lions and enemy tribesmen do not adhere to the idea of a 'comfort break' when they are in hot pursuit of you.

Once the challenge is over and it is safe to relax, your blood can flow back to your abdomen and digestion can start. This is the role of the parasympathetic nervous system (PSNS). This system ensures that you produce stomach acids and that saliva starts to flow again. Remember the dry mouth when you are frightened? That is the effect of the SNS becoming active. All your digestive enzymes are produced, pancreatic juice flows, bile is produced and available, the muscles of the lining of your digestive tract start to move (peristalsis), urine is prepared and you get, from time to time, the urge to get rid of wastes.

Parasympathetic (PSNS) dominant

The two systems cannot both be on at the same time; they are mutually exclusive. This means that if the test shows you to be parasympathetic (PSNS) dominant, you have a fairly active digestive system and are very good at digesting and processing food. Generally you do well on, and feel satisfied by a meat and fish-based diet with certain fruits and vegetables and only small amounts of grains. Your system needs and benefits from the challenge of considerable amounts of meat in your diet. Poultry choices should be for the dark meats rather than the light breast meat and fish will be less important to you than meat. You can feel unsatisfied if you have had a vegetarian meal or a meal of salads and fruits.

Sympathetic (SNS) dominant

If the test shows you to be sympathetic (SNS) dominant, it indicates that your metabolism is focused on activity, mental or physical, and the outside world, and less interested in digestion. You therefore generally have a less active digestive system and usually do well on a vegetarian diet with small amounts of fish. You can feel satisfied on a meal of salads or fruit, but you feel sluggish after a heavy meat meal, which taxes your digestion, perhaps giving you indigestion and leaving you feeling sluggish for hours as your limited resources struggle to digest it all. You will do much better on a vegetarian, or even a vegan, diet than one with lots of meat, which you should avoid, choosing fish instead if you want a 'meaty' meal. If you eat poultry, choose the light breast meat rather than the dark meat.

Note that whether you are SNS dominant or PSNS dominant, both systems will be working as appropriate. It is your emphasis that will vary.

Your test result will give you the lists of the foods that best suit your individual type.

Balanced autonomic

If the tests show you to be balanced autonomic, you can eat a wide range of foods; however, you will do best if, at any one meal, you choose foods that are appropriate for either one or the other of the two previous types. You have five groups of foods from which to choose: (a) those that are excellent if you decided to have a PSNS-type-diet meal (usually written in green); (b) those that are excellent for you if you decided to have a SNS-type-diet meal (usually written in purple); (c) those that are good for you (written in black); (d) those that you can eat occasionally (written in grey); and (e) those that you should avoid entirely (written in red and crossed through).

Cellular oxidation

If your results indicate that you fall within one of the last three categories, it indicates that your metabolism is based more on your rate of cellular oxidation (combustion) than your autonomic nervous system.

Fast oxidiser

If you are a fast oxidiser, you will burn food up rapidly. This again means that your system can deal easily with the challenge of meats and heavier meals. If faced with a meal of salad and fresh fruit you would burn it up almost as fast as you ate it and you would remain hungry and looking for something more. You are, therefore, similar to the parasympathetic dominant type described above.

Slow oxidiser

If your results indicate that you are a slow oxidiser, it indicates that you burn food up slowly. A meal of vegetables and fruit can satisfy you for a long time and you do not do well on a heavy meal of red meat. You are, therefore, similar to sympathetic dominant, above.

Balanced oxidiser or mixed oxidative

If you are balanced, in this case a balanced oxidiser, you will choose foods for each meal that come from either one or the other halves of your balance, from the fast oxidiser list or the slow oxidiser list.

Fine differences

Although it may sound as if the PSNS dominant and the fast oxidiser can eat similar foods, you will find, if you and some of your friends do the test, that there are subtle differences. The same is true for SNS dominant and slow oxidisers.

There is a second test option, and although it does not entirely jibe with the above, it is as valid, just as there are many different ways of slicing a sphere, yet they are all part of the same whole.

This test analyses the minerals found within a hair sample and is offered by Analytical Research Labs Inc. http://www.arltma.com and by Trace Elements Inc. www.traceelements.com, both in the US. The test results will give you information about your level of essential minerals, additional minerals, toxic elements and metabolically significant ratios. The analysis and report will also give you information on your metabolic type and some possible endocrine imbalances. The report comes with suggestions for the most appropriate foods and supplements to take. It costs slightly more than the previous test but provides considerably more information.

Metabolic typing may sound complicated, but my experience with countless patients is that many of them find that once they eat their correct diet, on this basis, they start to feel wonderful. Minor aches and pains, small problems, general feelings of malaise, all these start to disappear. Even when someone initially complains that they are being deprived of a favourite food, they come in time to realise that they are a lot better off without it and that they do not want it any more.

Simon D

One of my clients, Simon, was in his fifties, overweight, with high blood pressure and a severe lack of energy. He was concerned about cancer and assured me that he kept trying to stick to the 'right' diet. He tried to do as his wife and the magazines told him and to stick to fish and to eat more vegetarian meals, but it was difficult, and he just didn't feel good. He said he 'knew' that meats were bad for him but he felt much better when he ate them. I asked him to do the Metabolic Typing test. As I expected, he turned out to be a fast oxidiser, which meant that eating meat was good for him. It was good not only for his taste buds but for his health as well. He proved this when, with my encouragement, he went on to a meat and vegetable diet, with few or no grains or sugars – the diet he enjoyed. His weight came down, as did his blood pressure, and his energy level went up. Because of his concern about cancer he still ate relatively small portions of meat and large ones of vegetables. But whenever he felt he needed more meat he ate it.

Gerry Z

When Gerry came to see me, he had had a tumour in his colon removed but still had a small tumour in his prostate that was being watched. He wanted to know how he could assist all that he was doing with his doctor. He found that his metabolic type was SNS dominant and he improved his diet accordingly. He had always resisted giving up meat, as he frequently ate out in restaurants, entertaining clients, but soon learned to choose lighter meals and to select fish rather than meat. He took only a few of the supplements I recommended, aimed largely at making good some of the nutrient deficiencies indicated by his test results, and he started having daily coffee enemas (these are described in Chapter 15). I felt there was still a long way for him to go; he felt he had made sufficient changes. Certainly his general health improved, and even his PSA (the test for prostate cancer) started to come down. The future of his prostate cancer is unknown, but one of the pleasing results of what he had done was the improvement in his general health and the fact that his blood pressure had fallen sufficiently that he no longer needed his blood pressure medication.

A Blood-Type Diet

Some people like to work with a diet according to their blood type. If you know your type, whether it is O, A, B, or AB, it is temptingly easy.

However, it is not unknown for the diets indicated on this basis to contradict the diet indicated by your metabolic type. If this occurs, it is my experience that you would be well advised to stick to your metabolic-type diet.[21]

Food Quality

Poor-quality foods constitute another of the dietary predisposing factors. Once you have established the specific foods that are uniquely suited to you, it is time for you to focus on two other aspects of your dietary predisposing factor: a deficiency of good foods and an overload of bad foods. In general they occur together and we will consider both topics.

With regard to improving the quality, the first step is to buy organically produced and prepared food (see box on page 75). If you are really determined to do all you can to be healthy, you will buy foods only if they carry the organic label, or the equivalent in other countries.

A growing number of my patients make certain that all the food they buy is organic. On the other hand there are those people who criticise organic food either in terms of quality or cost. Certainly, there are different standards of organic foods, and maybe some of them leave something to be desired, but overall they are almost certainly somewhat better, and generally a lot better, than foods laden with a wide range of chemicals. They may or may not contain more nutrients, but they should certainly contain very much less in the way of a toxic or carcinogenic burden.

You may indeed occasionally find certain levels of pesticides in some organically produced foods. No farmer can stop the flow of air from neighbouring farms, or can control the level of chemicals in the rainwater or in the rivers flowing through their land. However, at the very least, organically grown and produced food is better than food that is produced with the intentional use of a variety of agricultural chemical additives and processed with more food additives.

The cost of organic food

You may argue that the cost of organically grown food is high yet, as more and more people choose it, the price comes down and it is often not that much greater than the cost of the commercially produced alternatives that use chemicals. If you think the commercial, bigger and cheaper lettuce looks like a better buy than the organically grown one, consider its water content. Many commercial foods seem bigger and heavier than their organic equivalents because of changes induced in their internal osmotic pressures (a detail that need not concern us here), which increases their fluid uptake. You are, in effect, buying water. If you are concerned that there is less weight of production of organically grown foods from an acre of land than there is of commercial foods, think about this weight issue and also consider eating less meat. It takes a lot more land to feed a family of carnivores than it does to feed a family of vegetarians, or even of partial vegetarians eating only small amounts of meat. If your metabolic type indicates meat as being good for you there is still no reason why you can't eat less of it and replace the rest with other recommended protein foods such as fish or nuts. It also costs less. Meat is expensive. You may find that some of your food budget is spent on unnecessarily expensive foods. Costly cakes and deserts can be more expensive than organic fruit. Potato crisps can cost more, for their actual nutrient content, than a few raw nuts.

Not all vegetables are equal

Whether organically grown or not, your food should be washed using some of the purpose-designed chemical-free vegetable washing liquids. In the main, try to buy foods that are still in the form in which they grew. This means, for instance, buying whole tomatoes rather than cans of tomato soup. You should avoid processed foods as much as possible; they provide hiding places for unwanted ingredients. These include such ingredients as sugar, white flour or vegetable oils (see box opposite), all of which are discussed below, even if they are organically produced.

If you decide to compromise somewhat, you could buy mostly organic foods, when you can, and other foods when they are not available from an organic source. In general, though not always, the foods in the health-food shops contain fewer additives and unwanted ingredients than regular supermarket lines. However, increasingly, you can buy these same foods at a lower price in some of the more enlightened supermarkets. Read the labels and be vigilant. Anything that carries E numbers or chemical terms with which you are not familiar should be avoided. A few E numbers refer to beneficial ingredients, even some of the vitamins, but in general if a vitamin is contained the manufacturers will be proud to say so; if it is a chemical with possible toxic effects they are more likely to hide behind the E number.

If you buy foods that have ingredients with names you do not recognise, put the names into a search engine and learn what you can about them, then decide if you are willing to eat them. It is no longer enough to assume that if the legislation allows their use they must be safe. We know this to be not true.

A word about terms

Organic To the informed chemist, the word 'organic' covers an enormous range of chemical compounds including most of the molecules in plants and animals and our own bodies, as well as many toxins such as petrochemical derivatives and many of the chemical food additives. Throughout this book the word is given the conventional meaning applied in this context. It is taken to mean anything that is approved by the associations that control organic farming and gardening and organic food production.

Vegetable oils As used in this book the term 'vegetable oils' covers oils such as sunflower, peanut, palm, corn and rapeseed (canola). They are commonly referred to as 'vegetable oils' on the label, particularly if a mixed oil is used. All may contain trans-fatty acids and other unwanted compounds produced in the manufacturing and processing procedures. When used in this pejorative sense the term does not include olive oil, coconut oil, flaxseed oil or hemp oil, all of which can be produced by safer methods and which have nutritional and health benefits.

The hidden carcinogens

Many agricultural and food additives are known carcinogens, or substances that can change into carcinogens within your body. An example of the latter is the nitrates that are added to a variety of foods such as so-called smoked meats and bacons. Although some smoked meats are truly smoked, many of them rely on such flavour enhancers to provide much of the flavour. This nitrate, on its own is not such a toxic substance. It certainly benefits the seller: it keeps the meat looking red and fresh, even if it isn't, and it imparts a more meaty and seemingly desirable flavour. Unfortunately, in the acid environment of your stomach, and in the presence of the proteins from the meat itself, the nitrates are converted into nitrosamines and these are carcinogens. Another example involves sodium benzoate; this is a permitted preservative in many foods and drinks including those containing acid fruits rich in vitamin C. Unfortunately, in addition to the side effects it can cause, when sodium benzoate combines with the vitamin C in the food, benzene is released and this is toxic.

You can avoid many food additives by buying fresh produce and preparing your own meals and sauces. This leaves you in greater control of what you eat. It may take a bit of time at the start, until you get used to doing this, but it can soon become a matter of routine.

All this may mean making some major changes to your current diet, but the good news is that by the simple actions you choose in relation to food choices, you can have a huge impact on your health and recovery, as Malcolm, above, did.

Good Foods

It is impossible to design a one-diet-fits-all protocol. However, some guidelines as to which foods are generally good and which should generally be avoided are given in the chart below.

It is a 'natural' and healthy eating programme aimed at giving you the maximum amount of benefit. The instructions are rigorous. There is little point in me making a half-hearted attempt to advise you on the best way to eat. If you choose to make your diet more liberal than this list indicates, that will be up to you, and may very well suit your circumstances. It is better to aim high and fall a little short than to aim low and achieve less. If you already have cancer you should follow these instructions, in their more restrictive form, rigorously. Make your food choices both according to the guidelines opposite and to your metabolic type. For instance, where it says you can eat all types of vegetables in the chart opposite, you will then choose those that are within your metabolic type list.

Foods to eat and foods to avoid

Food group	For prevention	If you have cancer or to avoid a recurrence	Avoid
General	All food should be organically grown and fresh. Frozen is occasionally acceptable	All food should be organically grown and fresh. Frozen is occasionally acceptable	Canned foods and highly processed foods
Vegetables	Almost all vegetables can be included. At least half of them should be eaten raw, including juices. The rest lightly steamed	Vegetables, including juices, should make up 75 per cent of your diet. Most of them should be consumed raw	Potato and parsnips (have a high glycemic index – see page 198). Canned vegetables. Fried vegetables or vegetable crisps, such as corn chips or potato crisps
Soups	Home-made soups, cooked for a minimum of time. Do *not* overcook	Vegetable soups made by blending raw vegetables and warm water (at body temperature)	Commercial or overcooked soups. Canned or packaged soups (using dry ingredients) unless organic or free from additives
Vegetables, fermented	Sauerkraut and other lactic-acid fermented vegetables	Sauerkraut and other lactic-acid fermented vegetables	Conventional pickles and chutneys with added chemicals and sugar
Fruits	Fresh fruits. The brightly coloured fruits are generally best. These are rich in a wide variety of phytonutrients. Lesser amounts of pale coloured fruits, such as pears, pale stone fruits, etc.	Only berries, they are high in vital nutrients and low in sugar. Frozen ones are acceptable if they cannot be obtained fresh	Bananas (contain sucrose – see page 97). Frozen fruit (other than berries). Canned fruit, sweetened fruit or fruits in syrup or with added sugar

Food group	For prevention	If you have cancer or to avoid a recurrence	Avoid
Dried fruits	Must be organic. Eat in small quantities. Fresh is better. Dates and goji berries can be used to sweeten biscuits and desserts	Goji berries if you must have something sweet. Other dried fruits are too sugar dense	Non-organic dried fruits contain toxic sprays to preserve them and their colour. Many are laxative. Contain large amounts of sugars
Fats and oils	Flaxseed oil (stored in the deep freeze, even after opening), hemp oil, olive oil, coconut oil. Occasionally butter if made from unpasteurised (raw) organic milk from grass-fed animals	Focus on flaxseed oil. Store it frozen, it melts within minutes at room temperature and can be used as normal	Other nut and seed oils. Vegetable oils. Commercial mayonnaise or salad dressings. Any fats containing trans-fatty acids. Animal fats, shortening, margarine and other alternative butter spreads. Rancid fats. Fats cooked to a high temperature
Soy	Fermented soy products, tempeh, miso, soy sauce (all organic)	Fermented soy products, tempeh, miso, soy sauce (all organic)	Non-fermented soy products, soya milk, tofu, textured soya protein products. The beans contain an anti-nutritive factor that inhibits the pancreatic enzymes that fight cancer cells
Beans and sprouts	Alfalfa, broccoli and other seeds and beans, sprouted. Beans can also be cooked	Alfalfa, broccoli and other seeds and beans, sprouted	Peanuts (strictly speaking these are a legume, not a nut), difficult to digest and may contain carcinogenic fungi
Nuts	Fresh raw nuts, ideally soaked first. Raw nut butters with no additions, freshly made in small quantities and kept refrigerated	Fresh raw nuts, soaked before eating. Raw nut butters with no additions, freshly made in small quantities and kept refrigerated	Peanuts. Fried, roasted or salted nuts and nut butters. Rancid nuts

Seeds and kernels	Chia, flaxseeds, pumpkin, sesame, sunflower or hemp seeds. Apricot, nectarine, peach and plum kernels, apple seeds. All raw	Chia, flaxseeds, pumpkin, sesame, sunflower or hemp seeds. Apricot, nectarine, peach and plum kernels, apple seeds. All raw	Roasted, fried or salted seeds, nuts and kernels
Seasonings	Fresh and freshly dried herbs and spices. Potassium chloride salt	Especially basil, chives, coriander, rosemary, garlic, ginger, parsley, cayenne, cinnamon, cumin, black cumin, turmeric, kelp	Salt, commercial sauces and flavourings. High salt seasonings. Those containing sugar or vegetable oils
Eggs	Organic, lightly boiled or poached. Raw egg yolks. Do not eat the whites raw, their avidin combines with biotin*, an essential nutrient, and prevents its absorption	Organic, lightly boiled or poached. Raw egg yolks. Do not eat the whites raw, their avidin combines with biotin*, an essential nutrient, and prevents its absorption	Fried, or scrambled eggs, omelettes. Oxidised cholesterol (from overcooked yolks) is no use to your body and a source of possible harm to your arteries. Commercial or free range eggs (unless also organic) in any form
Dairy	Organic buffalo, sheep or goat's yoghurt quark, kefir or small amounts of cottage cheese, possibly small amounts of hard cheese, preferably made from raw, unpasteurised, milk from grass-fed animals**	Organic buffalo, sheep or goat's yoghurt, kefir or quark. No other dairy products. Must be organic and raw for the best results. Should be blended with flaxseed oil	Pasteurised, homogenised or other processed milk. Commercial butter. Hard cheeses, cheese with more than 40 per cent fat

* Avidin is the protein in egg whites; biotin is the B-complex vitamin found in egg yolk.

** Ideally, all milk and cheeses, especially hard cheeses, should be avoided. There is growing awareness of the dangers of casein, the major protein in milk, in relation to cancer as was found in the Campbell study in 2004.[22] The study found that the researchers could 'switch cancer on and off' in two tissues (liver and breast) by giving experimental animals (rats and mice) four different carcinogens (aflotoxin, HBV, DMBA or 7,12-dimethylbenz(a)anthracine), NMU or N-nitroso-methylurea and then feeding the animals either a high casein diet (see box on page 82) or removing casein from their diet.

Food group	For prevention	If you have cancer or to avoid a recurrence	Avoid
Meat and fish	Meat and fish according to your metabolic type. Meat and poultry should be from organic, grass-fed animals	High omega-3 fish, organic salmon and other oily fish. Small amounts of fish, poultry and red meats depending on your metabolic type. Meat and poultry must be from organic, grass-fed animals	Smoked, salted, fried or processed meats or fish. Processed meats with any additives. Avoid nitrates, antibiotics, hormones, growth factors
Drinks	Generous quantities of fresh vegetable juices made from greens, carrots, beetroot, broccoli, celery, fennel, cabbage (dark green or red), kale, cress, etc., with ginger. Nut milks (without vegetable oils or sugar). Herb teas and green tea. Dandelion coffee. Water: 1 litre (1¾ pints) for every 22.7kg (3½ stone/50lb) body weight per day	Concentrate on juices from above-ground vegetables to avoid an excess of starch and sugars. Herb teas, green tea and pure water. Water: 1 litre (1¾ pints) for every 22.7kg (3½ stone/50lb) body weight per day	All soft drinks, carbonated drinks (including sparkling mineral water), fruit juice drinks, pre-made fruit juices, coffee, alcohol. Any drinks with sugar. Even fruit juices deliver too much sugar too quickly and without the fibre – eat the fruit instead. Avoid plastic containers
Cereals	Sprouted grains, wheat grass juice. Millet, buckwheat, brown rice, amaranth, quinoa	Avoid grains because of the high starch and glucose content	Wheat, white flour, white pastas, white rice
Breads	Rye, millet buckwheat, yeast-free breads, sprouted grain breads – unless told not to eat such high-starch foods.	Avoid grains	Wheat bread. Breads made with refined (white) flour

Sweets	Xylitol, ribose, mannose, stevia*. Lactitol, mannitol, maltitol and erythritol may be acceptable. (A few people may find that they cause mild diarrhoea.) They are found in some 'sugar-free' manufactured foods	Xylitol, ribose, mannose, stevia*. Lactitol, mannitol, maltitol, and erythritol may be acceptable. They are found in some 'sugar-free' manufactured foods	Sugars, under any name, in anything: sugar, evaporated cane juice, rice, maltodextrin, corn syrup, glucose, fructose, fruit sugar, agave, etc. All artificial sugar substitutes, saccharine, cyclamates, sucralose, aspartame, etc.
Miscellaneous	Carob powder. Pure organic cocoa powder	Carob powder. Pure organic cocoa powder	Commercial chocolates, sweets, lollies, sugar-laden 'health' bars

*Stevia is not currently available in the EU.

What is casein?

Casein is water-insoluble and makes up approximately 80 per cent of milk proteins. Whey proteins are water-soluble. When milk is made into cheese the water-insoluble casein goes into the curd, and so to the cheese, whereas the water-soluble whey proteins go into the liquid whey. Thus, powdered 'whey protein isolate', although it is derived from milk, is casein-free. If a product is simply labelled 'whey protein' there may be small amounts of casein in it if the extraction process has not been rigorous. 'Whey powder' contains not only the whey proteins but lactose or milk sugar as well, and this is undesirable on a sugar-free diet.

The situation regarding natural yoghurt, casein and cancer is less clear. Firstly, there is some suggestion that casein is changed structurally when yoghurt is made, secondly Dr Budwig (see page 101–2) claimed good results using yoghurt mixed with flaxseed oil in her anti-cancer diet. Some of my patients choose to use pea protein plus cysteine-rich whey protein, combined with the flaxseed oil, instead of yoghurt.

You will notice in the previous table that there is frequent mention of raw foods. These include all foods that are either completely raw or that have been slow-dried, as long they have never been heated to above 40°C (105°F). Heating foods above this temperature causes the breakdown of valuable enzymes whose benefit depends both on their composition and their shape. By using a dehydrator – a purpose-designed cabinet with accurate temperature controls – you can produce many interesting foods to add to your raw diet. (See Resources for sources of the dehydrator and for recipe books.)

The higher the proportion of raw foods in your diet the healthier it will be. If you are currently focused on prevention, you should aim to have two meals a day that are mostly raw and possibly add a side salad or some fresh fruit to the third. If you have cancer, you should aim for as high a raw content as you can manage. One hundred per cent raw would be wonderful, but most people settle for around 75 per cent.

If You Have Cancer

- You should avoid all fruits other than berries because of their high sugar content. Berries are rich in many beneficial phytonutrients, such as ellagic acid, and relatively low in sugar. Citrus fruit is acceptable provided you eat all the skin as well as the sweet centre. If this sounds strange, think of it as liquid marmalade. The nutrients in the skin compensate for the sugar in the juice. Try putting an entire orange and/or lemon (chopped) into a high-powered blender, along with fresh herbs, onions, garlic, vinegar and oil, to make a delicious salad dressing.

- Avoid dried fruit: it contains too much sugar. An exception could be small amounts of goji berries if you want a 'sweet snack'; combine them with raw nuts.

- At least 75 per cent of your food should be raw. This can include your juices, which helps.

- Either avoid all dairy products or limit them to the organic, and preferably unpasteurised, yoghurt or quark used in Budwig mixes (see pages 101–2).

- Avoid all grains; they are high in starch, which breaks down to glucose, they provide relatively few phytonutrients, and any moulds on them are generally toxic.

Keep in mind that these are guidelines and should be adjusted according to your metabolic type.

The Mediterranean Diet

You may feel the diet as dictated by your metabolic type and the Foods to Eat or Foods to Avoid table above is too restrictive, or that it may appear somewhat arbitrary. If you want a less rigorous and more general suggestion, one that is easier to live with but still healthy, then here it is: follow a Mediterranean diet. Note, however, that this is not the Mediterranean diet of Spain (which has too much white rice), France (which has too much white bread), or Italy (which has too much white-flour-based pastas). It is the Mediterranean diet of Crete soon after the

Second World War, when they were, partially by their own choice, essentially cut off from external food trade. It is easy to imagine the nature of the diet for yourself if you think of a Mediterranean island without any imports. This is meant as a dietary guide and not an absolute political or historical statement; however, these people at this time had exceptionally good health and the concept is worthy of attention.

This Mediterranean diet was based on local produce, largely grown naturally, without access to imported pesticides, hormones or other such chemical additives, which were not readily available. It was based on vegetables, fruits and local fish plus small amounts of meat, dairy products and eggs, largely unprocessed except in the kitchen. A relatively small number of sheep and cattle could be farmed on the island, and so meat intake was limited and came from grass-fed animals, not from, for instance, cattle that had been fed on corn and other grain-based concentrates. Dairy products were raw (neither pasteurised nor homogenised). Eggs came from what we would now call free-range and organic hens. Local honey, available in limited amounts, took the place of sugar. Olive oil, which can be extracted with relatively little processing, was used for salads and cooking.

Very little grain was grown in that climate and so played little part in the diet. Local grapes allowed for the production of wine and some brandy, but without imports the total alcohol consumption was limited. Most of the wine was red, incorporating skin and seeds, to get the most out of the grapes. Red wine is rich in protective compounds such as resveratrol and other salvesterols, which offer many benefits against cancer; white wine contains almost none of these. Given the climate of Crete it is easy to imagine that much of the food was eaten raw, as salads and fresh fruit. These suggestions make a good starting point if you want to change your diet slowly, and do it without a lot of rules or regulations as contained in the guidelines in the chart above.

Alkaline Diet

The moment you start to think of cancer and diet in the same context you will almost certainly think of, read about or be told about, the value of eating an alkaline diet. This is a diet that leaves an alkaline rather than an acid residue in your body. It does not relate to the acidity or alkalinity of the food itself, measured outside the body. In general, an alkaline residue diet is one that is rich in vegetables and fruits and contains minimal amounts of meats, fats and starches.

If your metabolic type is that of a slow oxidiser or you are sympathetic nervous system (SNS) dominant you are probably too acidic and will do best on an alkaline-residue diet, rich in vegetables and some fruits. If you have, or have had, cancer it is probable that your tissues are too acidic. It is also possible, though much less likely, that you are too alkaline, as cancer is thought to develop more readily in an acidic than in an alkaline body. If you are a fast oxidiser or parasympathetic nervous system (PSNS) dominant you may err on the side of being too alkaline and so do better on a more acid-residue diet, hence the suggestion that you eat more acid-residue foods such as meats. Be warned, however, that like all generalisations there are exceptions. These are just guides. Even if your results indicate the value of meats in your diet, if you are intent on avoiding or treating cancer you would be wise to include significant amounts of vegetables, for all the beneficial and anti-cancer nutrients they contain, and relatively smaller amounts of meat and fish because of all the additives and other toxins they can contain that have come from many different sources. These include the feedstuffs given to the animals in the form of concentrates and dry foods, chemicals added to their pastures and various veterinary treatments.

Why organic meat is better for you

This is a good time to make a further point about the value of choosing organic foods, particularly when it comes to eating large amounts of meat. Meat can carry a heavy load of toxins in the form of hormones, antibiotics, growth promoters and other chemicals that boost the production of the animal for the farmers. They also contain the additives in the feed concentrates and, if concentrates are fed instead of grass, an excessive amount of omega-6 fatty acids instead of the valuable omega-3 fatty acids (see Chapter 10). All this gives the farmer a better price but does nothing for your health and can put you at increased risk of cancer.

Combining the alkaline diet with metabolic typing

As most (although not all) people with carcinomas – the cancers that account for 80–90 per cent of solid tumours – are sympathetic dominant or slow oxidisers and are generally too acidic, it is easy to see how it has become an accepted mantra that people with cancer should eat an alkaline-residue diet. They need a diet rich in vegetables and with little or no red meat or poultry. This is not a hard-and-fast rule and is an early example of the importance of doing the tests, in this case the Metabolic Typing Test. You just might be one of those people who needs a more acidic-residue diet, so do the test, it is important to know what is best for you rather than going on assumptions and generalisations.

Testing Your pH

The alkalinity or acidity of anything – whether fruit juice or the state of your body – is measured by a number called the pH. pH is a measure of the pressure (or quantity) of hydrogen ions in a (watery) liquid. It is a reciprocal relationship, so the lower the pH figure the more hydrogen ions are present and the more acid is the solution. It is also a logarithmic relationship, so a pH of 7 is ten times more alkaline than a pH of 6. The pH can range from 1 to 14 and a neutral pH is close to 7.

There are many fluids in your body, such as the blood and lymph, and there are others that are produced by your body and secreted out of it, such as saliva and urine. There are desirable or normal pH values for all of them. If your pH is too low and you are too acidic, this is an early-warning sign that your health needs attention. By monitoring your pH and the way that it changes as you institute changes in your life, you can gauge the progress you are making towards better health.

In general, cancerous or unhealthy tissues are acidic, and healthy tissues are neutral to slightly alkaline. Remember, cancer thrives in an acidic environment. At pH 7.4 cancer cells hibernate, they cease to metabolise or to be active and grow. At pH 8 or above they start to die. Many of the successful CAM therapies that have been suggested for use in the treatment of cancer have, as part of their end result, whether intended or not, the effect of increasing the body's pH, of moving the body from acid to alkaline.

The ideal direct measurement would be to monitor the pH of your tissues, but this is difficult. The next best option would be to measure the pH of your blood. But blood is a complex fluid, with the pH varying from serum to plasma and to the cells within it. It is also buffered (maintained within normal limits, as far as possible) by a number of mechanisms, so in a sense it is not a particularly good guide to the general pH of your body. The more accessible fluids are those produced by your body, and both saliva and urine can give indirect indications of your tissue pH.

This pH monitoring is far from an exact science, but the pH of your saliva, first thing in the morning, before you have had anything to eat or drink, is thought to indicate the state of your tissues. Ideally, this pH reading should be neutral (pH = 7) to slightly alkaline (slightly above pH = 7). Saliva pH will rise when you are about to eat and will stay high for a short while after a meal. This is to aid digestion and because the digestive enzymes in your mouth, the starch-splitting amylases, work best at an alkaline pH. The initiation of eating, even only in thought, can stimulate the flow of this alkaline solution and the associated enzymes. So a pH measured immediately before or soon after eating is a function of digestion and does not mean that your tissues have suddenly become alkali. This is why the best time to get a background reading is early in the morning, before you have eaten.

Urine pH is thought to reflect both your diet and the way you have processed what you have consumed. If the diet is high in acid-forming foods, then your daytime urine pH should fall (become acid) as the kidneys process these acids and pass them out in the urine. If you have eaten large quantities of vegetables and little else, your urine pH will probably rise. The best time to get a true background reading is the second urine flow in the morning, preferably before eating or drinking.

Measuring your pH level

This test is inexpensive, easy to perform and can be done by you, on your own. It can be carried out on a regular basis and can provide useful background and generalised information.

The pH level can be measured using a strip of pH paper. This can be purchased from some chemists or suppliers of chemical equipment or from Enzyme Processes. This pH paper has been impregnated with a chemical solution that changes colour with the change in pH. The paper comes in a roll and a small piece can be torn off for each test. This is much less expensive than buying individual plastic sticks with a small amount of this paper stuck to the end, which are suitable for only one test or use. The colours will vary with the chemical used, but generally a pH of 5 will turn the paper yellow, indicating acid. As the pH rises towards 7 the colour of the paper will change from yellow to a yellow/green and finally to a full green. From pH 7 to pH 8 the colour changes from green to blue. A colour chart comes with the paper. There are other papers covering different pH ranges and with different colours when different dyes are used. So check any result you get with the colour chart that will be provided with your sample paper. Here is how to do it:

Step 1 On rising, first thing in the morning, wash your mouth out with plain water and spit it out. Do not clean your teeth. Wait about ten minutes and then spit some saliva onto the pH paper. Be careful when measuring saliva pH. You do not want to swallow the dye on the pH paper, so be sure to spit onto it, do not put it against your tongue. Write down the pH reading.

Step 2 Pass and discard your first morning urine, which will be influenced by the way your body processed the foods eaten during the previous day. Wait for an hour or so until you can pass a small amount of freshly formed urine. Measure the pH of this mid stream. The pH determined in this way reflects the state of your tissues when there is minimal dietary influence. Do not eat or drink until after you have made both of your measurements.

What the results tell you

The pH of healthy people is slightly alkaline, from 7.5 down to 7.1. People who are slightly less than ideally healthy have a pH range from 7.1 down to 6.5. People whose tissues vary from mildly to strongly deficient in alkaline minerals and who are probably heading in the direction of serious degenerative health problems, including the possibility of cancer, will generally find that their urine is between weakly acidic at a pH of 6.5 down to a strongly acidic pH of 4.5.[23]

Most children have a salivary pH of 7.5. About half the adult population has a reasonably healthy pH in the range 7.5 down to no less than 6.5 but that also means that half of all adults show a pH of 6.5 or lower. This latter is a reflection of the acid residues derived from the foods of commerce and the deficient intake of calcium and other minerals. It is associated with increasing age and ill health, particularly with degenerative diseases and cancer.[24] People with cancer often show an acid pH of 6 down to 4.5. Please note, however, that this is NOT a test for cancer, although the changes in pH may be found associated with it.

The relationship between the two figures is important. Most of the time, when you are in a healthy state, and when you eat a balanced diet consisting of the correct food for your body type, your saliva pH will be slightly higher than your urine pH. This is good.

If, in spite of all your good work and any efforts you have put into changing your diet, your saliva pH is low but your urine pH is high, it suggests that your tissues are too acidic. Your kidneys are not processing and removing the excess acids, and these acids are not being passed out in your urine; however, all the alkaline minerals you have been eating are being passed out in the urine. This is not good and you have further corrections to make.

If you are on a highly alkalising diet, such as a green juice fast, your urine pH may rise to 8 (the top level of many papers) or go beyond. This is all right as long as your saliva pH is also neutral to alkaline.

Getting your pH right, converting an acid system to a neutral or slightly alkaline one, is of vital importance if you are to improve your health and avoid or beat cancer.

There are many advantages to making sure your pH is neutral, even if you don't have cancer.[25] Most of the degenerative diseases occur when the pH is low and the body is acidic. These diseases include arthritis, tooth decay and osteoporosis, heart disease, and kidney and gallstones. To avoid them, raise your pH.[26]

Your Optimising Strategy

If your pH figures are too low, it's particularly important that you change your diet to one that is correct for you and that has more vegetables, some fruit and far fewer grain-based starchy foods and sugars, less fats and possibly less protein. If you want to raise your pH you should certainly eat fewer processed foods, such as those that fill most of the supermarket shelves other than the fruit and vegetable sections. This latter section is often the smallest in the supermarket, whereas in fact it should be the largest. This, on its own, is a sad testimony to the bad diet that most people eat. If your metabolic type indicates a meat-rich diet it will still include many different vegetables and very little starch or processed foods and, because of the way your body metabolises these foods, particularly the meats, this will be, for you, the appropriate diet.

You can help to flush unwanted acid residues out of your body by adding 100g of sodium bicarbonate (or baking soda not baking powder) to your bath water each day and relaxing in it for 20 minutes. Another method is to take 90 drops of d-lactic acid a day.

Food Sensitivities and 'Allergies'

Food sensitivities or allergies constitute another dietary predisposing factor. Many people have either (a) known food allergies; or (b) unsuspected food intolerances. The two are different. They can both be tested for and, if found, you should avoid the offending foods, at least until your immune system has improved. You should do this no matter what the state of your health. You should avoid these foods absolutely if you have cancer, as your immune system has its work cut out to deal with the cancer and you do not want to weaken it by challenging it needlessly.

If you suspect you have food allergies or sensitivities but are not sure, give yourself time before doing a test, as it may turn out to be unnecessary. Spend a month on your correct metabolic diet. This may in itself exclude the foods that don't agree with you – the foods to which you are sensitive. Alternatively, the diet may make you feel so good, and improve your health such that any sensitivities are no longer reactive. If you are still concerned about allergies or sensitivities, check them out. (Genova Diagnostics provide an excellent test, the FACT test – Food Allergenic Cytotoxic Test – see Resources.)

The two kinds of sensitivity differ in that:

1   **Food allergies**, or allergens, are generally obvious and a reaction occurs almost immediately after eating a specific food. You might, for instance, come out in hives every time you eat strawberries, or know that oysters cause a violent reaction. If you are truly allergic, as opposed to sensitive, to a certain food, you usually have an acute reaction to it and will know.

If you do have allergies you will have immune factors (antibodies) that can be detected in your blood, which respond to that food each time you eat it. When tested your blood may show an IgE antibody reaction to these foods. This is an allergic reaction and these foods are allergens. They generally persist long term.

2 **Food intolerances** are less obvious. Most people call these 'allergies' although this is not strictly accurate. Their effects are harder to detect and for this reason they are often known as masked food intolerances or sensitivities. (See my book *Living with Allergies* for a full discussion of this topic.)

Their effects can be devastating. You may, for instance, be sensitive to wheat or dairy products but not know it, or not relate this to such symptoms as persistent or frequent headaches, irritability, mental confusion or other general symptoms.

The FACT test is made using a blood sample. A drop of your blood is combined with a drop of each food solution. Your white blood cells, which are normally relaxed and relatively inactive, may show a tendency to attack certain foods. Many years ago this test was carried out by observing the reaction of the white blood cells under a microscope. Now the test involves measuring the chemical reaction that occurs when this reaction takes place.

Nutrients Versus Calories

Before we leave the topic of foods in general, there is one further important concept that we need to discuss and that is the caloric 'cost' of the beneficial nutrients you obtain. The story is far from this simple, but the following description will give you the general idea.

Let's assume that your body needs 2,000 calories of food a day. If you eat something that contains or releases 200 calories of energy, then it should provide at least 10 per cent of your nutritional requirements in terms of the macro- and micronutrients it contains. You can, for instance, get all your protein requirements from nuts or brown rice, but you would have to eat a lot more than 2,000 calories of them to achieve this and you would still not have satisfied all your vitamin and mineral requirements. So we talk of 'nutrient dense' foods. These are those foods that supply a generous amount of essential nutrients in relation to the number of calories they contain. You need to be aware of this when looking at some foods tables; for example, the foods that contain the most of a certain nutrient. You should look for the food that gives you the greatest amount of the nutrient *per calorie*, not per gram. Unfortunately almost all books list foods in the latter way.[27] This is why I wrote *What's in My Food?* in 1988. Not all foods provide all nutrients, so some will have to provide more than their share of proteins; others will provide more than their share of vitamins. They will then compensate for each other.

This chapter has been about foods, it is time now to move on to a discussion of the macro food components, such as the individual proteins, fats and carbohydrate.

CHAPTER 10

Predisposing Factor No. 2 – Macronutrient Errors

You eat for a number of reasons. Most obviously you eat for satisfaction, because you are hungry, for enjoyment of the food itself and for the social occasions that accompany it. In fact you rely on the food you eat for the essential substances you need to rebuild and repair old tissues and to provide the functional compounds such as hormones, neurotransmitters, enzymes, immune factors and more. Finally, you eat for energy, both cellular energy and whole body energy.

To achieve these goals your diet consists of macro- and micronutrients. The macronutrients include proteins, fats, carbohydrates, fibre and water, and are the subjects of this chapter. The micronutrients include vitamins and minerals, plus phytonutrients or plant compounds, which exert a beneficial effect on the body. There are many hundreds of these, and possibly thousands.

We can divide this predisposing factor – macronutrient errors – into two parts: deficiency of the specific macronutrients your body needs, and an excess of the ones your body does not need or that do it harm.

Your diet may be deficient in adequate amounts of some or all of the 20 different amino acids that you derive from protein foods; it may be deficient in the essential fatty acids, in fibre or in water. On the other hand, you may be eating nutrient-poor foods, such as refined (white) flour and related products, sugars and most saturated fats (coconut oil is a noticeable exception, as is organic butter in very small amounts). Specifically bad foods (in addition to being nutrient poor) are sugars and foods with a high glycemic index (explained in Chapter 17), most vegetable oils (excluding flaxseed oil, olive oil, coconut oil and hemp oil) and processed fats with their altered fatty acids, often in the form of trans-fatty acids but including other harmful products produced by their heating and processing.

It is important that you give your body all that it needs, and nothing that it does not need or that can harm it, if you are to prevent or fight cancer successfully. It is also important to eat foods that are highly nutrient dense.

Proteins

Proteins are made up of 20 different amino acids, all of which are essential and must be available in the correct proportions if you are to make all the proteins your body needs. Think of a belt made of coloured beads. To follow the pattern you have to have beads of all the right colours in the correct proportions and sequence. As soon as you run out of one of the colours you have to stop making the belt, or spoil the pattern. Body protein cannot have a spoilt pattern, so when you run out of one of the amino acids protein building stops, at least until that amino acid is supplied by the next meal.

Your liver is able, at least to some extent, to convert some of the amino acids into others by rearranging the components, but it can make only half of them in this way and not always in sufficient quantity. These are the so-called 'non-essential' amino acids. They are non-essential in the diet because your liver can make them provided it has all the needed components (usually amino groups from other amino acids you have eaten in more generous amounts), but they are essential for your body and for your health. This is an important point to understand.

Ten of them cannot be made in your body and so are absolutely essential in your diet. You simply have to eat them, or you become protein deficient. You have run out of one of the essential coloured beads and protein building has to stop at that point.

Animal versus vegetable

Contrary to much popular belief, all protein foods, with the exception of gelatine (an animal protein) contain all the amino acids; however, their proportions vary. In general, animal proteins contain a greater proportion of the essential-in-the-diet amino acids than do plant proteins. If you eat sufficient plant proteins, however, you can certainly get all your protein requirements.

The Optimal Nutrition Evaluation test, or ONE test offered by Genova Diagnostics

The ONE test, already mentioned, is a comprehensive test that assesses fundamental cellular function. It does not evaluate directly the quantities of nutrients in your diet or analyse the amounts in your body. Instead it provides an assessment of your cellular function, how good it is and where there may be any possible inadequacies. Based on this it is possible to determine indirectly any probable nutrient deficiencies and the possible presence of some toxins (by their consequences, such as slowing down a particular reaction). This means that the results of the test are specific to you and the way your body responds to the diet you have chosen.

The results obtained will provide the following information:

- A number of possible deficiencies: antioxidants, minerals, vitamins and amino acids.
- The state of your digestive tract: mal-digestion, inadequate protein absorption and inappropriate nitrogen balance, the presence of pathogens including yeasts and fungi.
- Your detoxification efficiency.
- Your level of oxidative stress and whether or not you need more antioxidants.
- Methylation deficiencies, and hence the risk of a number of diseases including cancer and heart disease.
- Neurotransmitter imbalances, and hence a multitude of problems, as these compounds carry instructions to almost every cell in your body.
- Energy production, by measuring the levels of the many components in the Krebs cycle (as explained in Chapter 16).

The test is carried out using a urine sample and is one that is referred to frequently throughout this book. It is well worth doing this as a basic test in relation to your general health.

How is your amino acid status?

A useful test to determine your amino acid status is the Optimal Nutrition Evaluation or the ONE test described above. The results from this test often show that people are deficient in some of the essential-in-the-diet amino acids, suggesting dietary deficiencies, or even in some of the not-essential-in-the-diet amino acids, suggesting that these amino acids are not being produced fast enough within your body, usually in your liver. If tests show you to be deficient in any amino acids, these deficiencies should be made good either by changing your diet or taking the appropriate supplements. The details as to what is needed and in what quantity will normally be provided by the test report.

The type of protein you should eat will be determined by your unique metabolic type, as discussed in Chapter 9. It is important that you follow the guidelines you receive with that report. I then advise that you do the ONE test to determine your own individual needs. You may well find that you are currently deficient in a number of amino acids.

The following calculation is for the non-existent 'average person', but can act as a rough guide for you until you determine your own unique needs:

Take your weight in pounds, and divide this by two.

That is about the weight of protein, in grams that you need.

Thus, if you weigh 10 stone or 140lbs you would need about 70g (2½oz) of protein a day.

Note that this does not mean you need only 70g (2½oz) of meat or fish. If the fish contained approximately 20 per cent protein and it was the only protein-containing food you ate, you would need to eat 350g (12oz) of it. In fact, of course, you will get various proteins from a wide range of foods.

Carbohydrates

Carbohydrates consist mainly of starches and sugars. The starches such as those in fruits, vegetables, legumes (beans, peas and lentils), grains and a few fruits are composed of branched chains of thousands of glucose molecules joined together. These chains are broken down within your digestive tract and eventually enter your bloodstream as glucose. Sugars are variable. Sucrose, or table sugar, for instance, is a double molecule, or dimer, made up of glucose joined to fructose. Similarly, lactose or milk sugar is a dimer of glucose joined to galactose. Most fruits contain fructose; bananas are an exception and contain sucrose. Honey contains glucose and fructose as separate molecules.

Fructose and galactose are absorbed and travel to your liver where they are converted into glucose. Thus the end product of most of the starches and sugars you eat is glucose. This glucose travels through your bloodstream and enters your cells. It does this with the help of insulin, zinc, chromium, vanadium, several B-group vitamins and a number of other nutrients.

Your present diet will almost certainly contain a sufficient quantity of carbohydrate; however, you may be eating the wrong type. Your carbohydrate intake should be mainly in the form of the complex carbohydrates from vegetables, as these also provide a wide range of other phytonutrients. In fact, in general, vegetables are the most nutrient-dense foods in terms of providing you with the essential minerals and vitamins and a wide range of cancer-fighting phytonutrients. In other words, you can eat a diet with large amounts of vitamins and minerals and yet not gain weight if you focused solely on vegetables. They provide the most nutrients per calorie.

Carbohydrates at a glance

Monosaccharides are single sugars, such as glucose, fructose, galactose, ribose and deoxyribose. Glucose is found on its own in honey, attached to fructose in sucrose, to galactose in the lactose found in milk and to another glucose molecule in maltose found in many confectionery products. It is attached to a large number of other glucose molecules in the starches and cellulose of most plant foods. Fructose, on its own, is found in honey and many fruits. Ribose and deoxyribose are part of RNA and DNA respectively and so found in flesh foods and in seeds. Ribose may also be found as a sweetener in some products. It can be obtained as a powder from some heath-food suppliers.

Disaccharides are double sugars, such as:
Sucrose (table sugar) = glucose–fructose
Lactose (milk sugar) = glucose–galactose
Maltose (from grains) = glucose–glucose
(**Note** honey contains glucose and fructose as free monosaccharides)

Starches are thousands of glucose molecules joined together by bonds that can be broken down within your digestive tract. They are made by, and found in, plants foods such as vegetables, grains and legumes.

Glycogen is thousands of glucose molecules joined together by bonds that can be digested within your digestive tract. It is made in animal and human cells.

Cellulose is thousands of glucose molecules joined together by bonds that cannot be broken down within your digestive tract. It is found in plant foods, particularly vegetable and whole grains and whole grain products, such as brown rice and wholemeal flour. It is one type of 'fibre' and not found in white flour or white rice, or in animal products.

Sorting through the grains

If you do not have cancer, small amounts of carbohydrate can come from true whole grains or their products. These include brown rice, rolled oats (not processed porridge oats) or wholemeal flour. It is probable, however, that you are eating too much of your carbohydrates in the form of refined carbohydrates such as white flour, white rice or white pasta and 'pretend' wholemeal breads (see below) and these should be excluded from any diet if you want maximum health. Check the list of ingredients on the packaging, the only grains listed should be wholemeal flour or, as appropriate, whole rye, and so on.

There are many such 'pretences'; they include breads that are slightly brown in colour, possibly due to the presence of some (but not all) wholemeal flour, or coloured substances such as malt (sugar). They may contain wheat meal, which is not the same as wholemeal, or carry such phrases as 'made from the goodness of whole country grains'. White flour comes from whole country grains, it has just had all the fibre and most of the vitamins and minerals, the goodness, removed from it and some type of bleach added to make it white.

A lot more of your carbohydrate intake probably comes from a variety of simple sugars. All of these are bad for you. They are bad if you think you are currently still healthy; they are a major threat to your recovery if you have cancer.

There are many reasons for consuming whole grain products rather than refined ones. Here are some of them:

- You will get all the nutrients that the grains contain but which are lost in processing, including many trace minerals and most of the B-group vitamins.
- You will eat the fibre that helps to prevent constipation, nourishing the cells that line your intestines, feeding the beneficial bacteria in your digestive tract and helping to remove toxins from your body (see Chapter 15.) Although this is true, the best fibre actually comes from vegetables, which contain an even wider range of beneficial nutrients. You can, if so advised, do without grains at all in your diet.
- Eating whole grains slows down the release of glucose from the starches and thus avoids the sudden surge in your blood glucose level that occurs after eating refined grain products.
- You will avoid the intake of refined, or high-glycemic, foods (discussed in Chapter 17).

There are many reasons for avoiding the simple sugars, as you will discover in Chapter 17. Put simply, sugar, and other high-glycemic foods, feed cancer.

In relation to carbohydrates, this predisposing factor comprises both a deficiency of vegetables and an excess of sugars and refined carbohydrate foods.

Fats

The majority of fats, more correctly called lipids, in your diet are used for energy. They are made of a variety of fatty acids, any three of which can be combined with glycerol to make a triglyceride, the common form found in food and in your bloodstream.

Other lipids are functional compounds with specific roles to play. They include such things as cholesterol, the lecithins or phospholipids, steroid hormones, specific brain and nerve cell fats and the essential-in-the-diet fatty acids that are vital components of cell membranes and lead to the production of compounds called prostaglandins.

Milk and calcium

There is often confusion in regard to the role of milk and its desirability as a source of calcium. Babies need large amounts of calcium and phosphorous for rapid bone building and so maternal milk (*of the same species)* is the ideal food. In fact cows' milk is significantly different from human milk in this regard, containing roughly twice as much calcium. This is hardly surprising, given the growth rate of calves. Milk is a much less desirable food for adults. In relation to the amount of calcium it contains there is too much phosphorous and far too little magnesium, which can encourage the loss of calcium in the urine. Better sources of calcium are many vegetables, such as cabbage, parsley, various seaweeds, endive, chard and celery, which have a similar amount of calcium per calorie to milk, but a much higher amount of desirable magnesium and less phosphorous. If you do chose to derive some of your calcium from dairy products then they should be full cream dairy products to maximise the calcium absorption, which needs the medium- and short-chain fatty acids found in milk.

The most common food lipids are the triglycerides and their many different fatty acids, two of which are essential because your body cannot make them. Many of the fatty acids are saturated, some are either mono- or polyunsaturated. Contrary to popular opinion, the saturated fatty acids are not all bad, some of them are important for your health. These are the short-chain saturated fatty acids such as those found in butter, and which assist the absorption of calcium, and the short- or medium-chain-length fatty acids found in coconut oil that are anti-fungal, anti-bacterial and anti-viral.

The omegas

Of the unsaturated fatty acids there are three important groups, namely the omega-3 group, the omega-6 group and the omega-9 group. The omega-3 and the omega-6 groups include fatty acids that are essential in the diet. The omega-3 group includes alpha-linolenic acid or ALA, which is essential in your diet. Other omega-3 fatty acids include EPA and DHA. The omega-6 group includes linoleic acid or LA, which is also essential in your diet, but also other omega-6 fatty acids that are not. These include GLA, DGLA and arachidonic acid or AA. They can be made in your body from the two essential fatty acids.

The essential fatty acids reside mainly in your cell membranes. They help to maintain healthy and flexible membranes around your cells and the internal organelles within the cells. Healthy membranes can easily house all the necessary receptor sites (usually proteins), which act as either locations or channels at, or through, which nutrients and information molecules are received or taken in, and through which information molecules, products of cellular activity such as hormones, and waste products leave the cell.

It is vital for good health that you have the correct amounts and ratios of polyunsaturated fatty acids and the healthy cellular membranes that result. This enables proper and efficient inter-cellular communication and metabolism. Whole books have been written on this subject.[28] Cell membranes can also act as storage locations for the essential fatty acids available for prostaglandin production.

Beneficial flaxseed oil

In this book we are focusing on tests. If you don't want to do these, to determine your fatty acid status, at the least make sure your diet includes a generous amount of flaxseed oil. Use this in salad dressings and in the Budwig mix (see below). Do not cook with flaxseed oil and do keep it in the deep freeze once the bottle has been opened. This will reduce the risk of it oxidising. It will melt rapidly when you want to use it, just hold the bottle in the warmth of your hands or under some warm water for a minute.

The Budwig mix Dr Joanna Budwig was an authority on fatty acids and was seven times nominated for a Nobel Prize. She advocated the use of a combination of flaxseed oil and organic quark or yoghurt. This, she stated, will optimise the fatty-acid content of your cell membranes and so max-imise cellular communication, improve cellular energy and reduce the risk of developing cancer (primary or from recurrence). She suggested a mixture of 30ml (2 tbsp) of flaxseed oil combined with 60ml (4 tbsp) of yoghurt, blended thoroughly for 60 seconds and allowed to stand for ten minutes. This, she stated, should be eaten three times a day.[29]

The rest of her diet is relatively liberal and allows significant amounts of honey, which is now considered a danger, as we know sugar feeds cancer.[30]

The role of prostaglandins

A second reason why we need the two essential fatty acids and their products relates to the groups of compounds they produce, called prostaglandins. Prostaglandins are vital communication and functional molecules at the cellular level, somewhat analogous to hormones at the organ level. In fact, it is simplest if you think of prosta-glandins as micro hormones. They are made almost on the spot where they are required, then act and break down almost immediately in response to cellular and chemical messages. As a result of their location, the prostaglandins can be made and dispatched rapidly as and when the cells are informed that they are needed. Here is a typical example: at the capillary level the blood fluid and its contents of mil-lions of cells is flying around your circulation system at high speed, the cells all jostling each other and bombarding the blood vessel walls as they fly by. The natural tendency, the moment there is a 'bump', is for a clot to form. To prevent this, immediately following each 'bump', a tiny amount of anti-clotting prostaglandin is pumped out saying, 'Don't clot!', and the blood flows smoothly on. The number of such 'bumps' and 'Don't clot! messages per second is almost unbelievably large. Without prostaglandins we would all suffer from immediate thrombi.

Prostaglandins perform hundreds of other such reactions that ensure you stay healthy. There are three groups of prostaglandins, which are well recognised:

1   The **omega-6 fatty acids** can be converted into a number of compounds known as the 'prostaglandin one group' or series – the PG1 series.

2 Similarly, **the omega-9 fatty acids** can be converted into prostaglandins of the two series, PG2.

3 And the **omega-3 fatty acids** are converted into prostaglandins of the three series, PG3.

The details are complicated and need not concern us here. In general the PG1 series are mildly clotting and anti-inflammatory, the PG2 series are strongly pro-clotting and highly inflammatory and the PG3 series are strongly anti-clotting and anti-inflammatory.

'Thrombotic' and 'inflammatory' may sound like actions you do not want. Certainly, you do not want an *excess* of either of those actions; however, you do want to form blood clots when you have cut yourself, and inflammation is part of your body's total defence mechanisms when, for instance, bacteria have invaded a wound. Equally, it is the highly prothrombotic nature of arachidonic acid that gives meat (rich in this fatty acid) a bad name in relation to potential heart attacks particularly for the slow oxidisers and SNS dominant metabolic types. Many types of fish, which are generally rich in the fatty acids that lead to the PG3 series, are helpful in avoiding heart attacks due to the antithrombotic nature of their fatty acids. See the table below.

Fatty acids and the prostaglandins

	Omega-3	Omega-6	Omega-9
Sources	Mainly fish, flaxseed oil, evening primrose oil, borage oil	Mainly plant seeds including evening primrose and borage	Mainly meat and poultry
Prostaglandin	PG3	PG1	PG2
Actions	Antithrombotic, anti-inflammatory	Mildly thrombotic and mildly inflammatory	Strongly thrombotic and strongly inflammatory. The source of many cytokines (see Chapter 22)
Essential fatty acid	Alpha linolenic acid ALA	Linoleic acid, LA	
Other fatty acids	EPA, DHA	GLA, DGLA	Arachidonic acid AA

Avoiding communication breakdown

Health requires good communication and function of your cellular membranes. Cancer cells prefer to isolate themselves, often even producing a protein coating to wall themselves off from healthy cells. Their membrane can be 15 times as thick as that of healthy cells. By understanding the role of these fatty acids and their importance for cellular communication, you can come to understand why it is important that you have the proper balance of them in your diet and in your tissues.

Yet another reason for eating organic products, especially organic animal products, relates to the types of fatty acids they contain as a result of organic farming practices. Most organically farmed animals are grass fed, whereas non-organically farmed animals are more often fed on a variety of concentrates. Grass-fed animals have healthier levels of the most desirable saturated fatty acids with the right chain lengths, and of the omega-3 essential fatty acids in particular, than animals that have been fed on concentrates.

That covers the first half of the lipid aspect of this predisposing factor: failing to obtain sufficient of the desirable fatty acids in your diet. The other half involves eating the wrong types of fats.

The Danger Fats

The fats that you don't need are the overheated and processed fats. Oils that have been extracted from soft sources such as olives and coconuts, and oils that have been carefully extracted from soft seeds such as flaxseeds can be extracted without doing them much damage. Oils that have been extracted from hard seeds such as sunflower seeds, corn kernels, peanuts, and so on, however, are either extracted using toxic solvents or they are extracted by applying high pressures, the so-called 'cold pressed' oils. The act of applying these high pressures generates such heat that the residual solids left behind are charred or burned and the oil is adversely affected. These seed oils contain a significant proportion of unsaturated fatty acids. This means they can be readily oxidised, a process that is accelerated by heat. When this oxidation occurs, toxic and carcinogenic compounds such as malondialdehyde are produced. This is an important reason for avoiding the majority of vegetable oils.

Heating nearly all fats tends to denature them or alter their structure. When heating up to the temperature just before butter *starts* to brown, the damage is relatively mild, but with increasing temperature the damage to the fats, and hence the risk to your health if you consume them, rises exponentially. This means that foods cooked in deep-fat fryers should be avoided, so should crisps, chips, the outer burnt fats on roasted meats and burnt crackling on the fat of a roast. In fact, the best way to cook meat is by long, slow cooking in a casserole or stew pot. Roasted nuts should be avoided as, despite their name, they are often deep-fat fried.

Fibre

Although fibre might seem like an uninteresting food, it plays a vital role in your digestive tract and is a major contributor to good health. Fibre, despite its name, is not actually or necessarily fibrous. Most foods that we call fibrous contain long-chain complexes of glucose and other carbohydrates that are bonded together by bonds that cannot be broken down by the digestive enzymes within the human digestive tract. As such, they should really be called 'non-digestible carbohydrates'. Cellulose, described above, is one type of fibre, others include lignins, pectin and chitin. These fibres traverse the length of your digestive tract intact until they arrive in your colon. Here the fibre performs a variety of functions:

- It provides a food source for many of the bacteria present which do have the enzymes to break the fibre down and so to release the glucose and other sugars that they contain. In a healthy digestive tract the bacteria that are present are beneficial and essential for life, so feeding them is important.

- Some of the fibre breaks down to produce a compound called butyrate which protects the cells lining your colon.

- The fibre provides bulk to increase the mass of material in the colon. This bulk then presses on the walls of your colon and stimulates the peristaltic action that pushes the contents along, so preventing constipation.

- Fibre holds water in the waste material. By keeping this mass moist it helps to add further to the bulk that stimulates peristaltic action and assists you to have three soft and easy bowel motions a day.
- By these various means the presence of fibre helps to reduce fermentation and putrefaction within your digestive tract.
- The waste material may contain a number of toxins, either from your diet or produced by your body and expelled by your liver. Any undigested carbohydrate that remains intact can absorb toxins and carry them out with it. Further, by reducing stasis and the risk of constipation, the toxins are rapidly expelled from your body, and the risk of re-absorption is reduced.

The best fibre comes from vegetables. This is followed by grain fibre. Since, in general, vegetables are also more nutrient dense than grains, this makes vegetables even more important in your diet.

Water

It is variously said that your body is between 60 and 90 per cent water. It all depends on what you include as 'water'. Whatever the figure, the fact remains that your body needs an adequate amount of water, daily, to be truly healthy. You need water to replace the daily losses that occur:

- During urination.
- In your stool.
- Via your lungs as you exhale.
- Via your skin when you sweat.
- Via your skin, continuously and 'insensibly'. Although this can be considerable, you are almost unaware of it.

The average commercially produced diet as eaten by most people consists mainly of relatively 'dry' foods, such as breads, sugars, meats and fats. It is then suggested that you should drink about 1 litre (1¾ pints) of water for every 25kg (4 stone/55lb) of body weight. If your diet is composed essentially of fresh fruits and vegetables you may need less, but probably not much less. You might argue that if you are not thirsty then you don't need to drink any more, but it seems that in this regard many people's thirst mechanism is faulty and has learned to adjust to a lower than healthy intake.

Ideally, you should drink fresh, pure water. Sadly most tap water is not pure and it is generally better to drink purified water or still mineral water. This should be stored in glass bottles rather than plastic ones, which can release a number of toxic compounds into the water, such as phthalates. You can also include in the total such drinks as herb teas, vegetable juices and clear soups. Tea, coffee and alcohol do not count, as they are diuretic and only further increase your need for water. Include fresh fruit juices if you do not have cancer, but if you do have cancer, or have had cancer, these contain too much sugar.

The fluids that you should not be drinking include coffee, alcohol, soft drinks and others that contain sugars, colouring and flavouring agents, fizzy drinks and colas. Many people find giving up alcohol to be asking too much. If you do, then reduce your intake to no more than two glasses of red wine a day. As mentioned earlier, at least you are then getting the benefits of some of the phytonutrients in the red grapes to offset some of the damage done by the alcohol.

Testing for the Vital Signs

There are many tests you can do in relation to this predisposing factor.

1. For protein and amino acids

The amounts of the different amino acids can be analysed in a urine sample. The working levels within your body are indicated, both directly and indirectly, by such tests as the ONE test (explained on page 95). This test is offered by Genova Diagnostics who will send you the appropriate kit with instructions as to how to collect the urine sample and then send it to them.

2. For fats and fatty acids

The ONE test and others can also give you indirect information as to your levels of the different important fatty acids. In addition you can request a specific fatty acid profile. This test, offered via Nutri-Link, is carried out on the red blood cells in a blood sample and it measures the levels of over a dozen different fatty acids in the cell membranes. The cell membrane is where most of the important fatty acids reside and it plays a major role in the way cells behave, so levels of the different fatty acids here can be critically important for your health. The report that comes with your results will generally explain them and tell you of which fatty acids you have too much, which you have too little, and what you can do to make appropriate corrections.

3. For carbohydrates

Carbohydrate tests relate mainly to glucose levels and are discussed in Chapter 17 where a fuller explanation is more appropriate.

4. For fibre

You should be having as many bowel motions in a day as the number of meals that you eat. For most people this means three meals and so should mean three bowel motions. If you are not, you are almost certainly not eating sufficient fibre or drinking sufficient water.

5. For water

This is a rough estimate rather than an accurate test, but it's worth trying. Pinch some of the skin on the back of your hand and lift until it forms a ridge. Let go. It should immediately return to lying fully flat. If any ridge remains, even for a second, you are probably dehydrated. You can compare this by pinching your skin somewhere else on your body, say your arm, where it will generally return to a flat surface very much more rapidly.

Your Optimising Strategy

If deficiencies of the essential amino acids are indicated, the first thing to do is to consider whether or not you have adequate protein in your diet. If not, if you increase your total protein intake you may correct the problem. If that doesn't solve the problem you may want to consider taking supplements for the missing amino acids. The report you get back, after doing the ONE test, will generally indicate the appropriate quantities to take.

If your results suggest deficiencies of the essential fatty acids, you should change your diet to correct this. It may mean increasing your dietary intake of oily fish or of plant oils such as flaxseed oil, evening primrose oil or borage oil, or it may mean choosing hemp oil, or eating more avocados and nuts. What you need to do will depend on both the fatty acids in which you are deficient and on your metabolic type. If you prefer, you can take these fatty acids in supplement form, as oil-filled capsules.

There is almost no chance that your diet will be lacking carbohydrates unless you are obsessed with dieting and you eat less than 60g (2⅛oz) a day. Doing this is almost always unhealthy and generally leads to nausea and ketosis (the presence of ketones such as acetone, detectable by its smell, in your urine). If you are eating such small amounts you should increase your intake of vegetables to bring your carbohydrate intake levels up to a healthy level. Tests can show you how well your body is handling them, and these are described in Chapter 16.

This chapter has considered the macronutrients, the proteins, fats and carbohydrates. We have also mentioned fibre and water. In addition, we could include air and I use this opportunity to remind you to breathe deeply – and not just from the top of your lungs – and to do so all the time. Now it is time to move on and consider the micronutrients, the vitamins, minerals and other phytonutrients.

CHAPTER 11

Predisposing Factor No. 3 – Vitamin Deficiencies

Vitamins are small organic molecules that are essential for health but cannot be made in your body and so must be obtained from your diet. This is a simple definition and needs some explanation and expansion:

- Although the above is true for most vitamins, vitamin D_3 can actually be made in your body, provided you have sufficient exposure to sunlight and that your kidneys and liver are healthy, as they are part of the synthesising process. This is better than the synthetic or plant-derived vitamin D_2 that is used in supplements.

- Biotin, sometimes thought of or considered to be a vitamin of the B complex, is essential for life, but although a small amount is obtained from your diet, the majority is made by bacteria in your small intestine. Thus you can become biotin deficient if you take antibiotics and so kill these bacteria. You can also become biotin deficient if you eat raw egg whites, which combine with the biotin in situ and prevent its absorption, in which case it is lost in your stool.

Protective substances

'Essential for life' is not quite the same thing as 'essential for robust good health'. There are many substances, mostly phytonutrients (found in plants) that greatly improve your health and the length and quality of your life, even though you might not die without them. They are protective substances, and without them you would almost certainly succumb to a variety of life-threatening health problems more readily than if you have included them in your diet. In this group we can include a variety of bioflavonoids that work with and add to the activity of vitamin C, and the various carotenes that both convert to vitamin A and have valuable attributes of their own. There are countless other protective substances, such as the curcumin found in turmeric, various active ingredients in garlic, the ellagic acid of raspberries and the resveratrol found on ripe grape skins. If you do an Internet search on any of these substances and add the word 'cancer' you will find a wealth of information, far more than can be included here. If you find all the information somewhat overwhelming and difficult to assess, this is where your practitioner should be able to help you.

The question of quantity is also important. Various levels of vitamins can be quoted and it is important that you understand their significance. There are a number of points to consider:

1   There is a level of intake below which an individual might die.

2   There is a level of intake below which serious deficiency signs might develop.

3   There is a level of intake below which mild malaise might occur with no specific symptoms, but simply a lack of total good health.

4   Finally, there is a level of intake at and above which the individual will feel supremely well.

Clearly you would want to take an amount that equates to the final point; however, the levels found on most supplement containers as being the 'Daily Requirement' is generally somewhere between points 2 and 3. The situation is further complicated by the fact that individuals' needs vary widely, some people needing as much as ten times as much of a particular nutrient as others. This is why testing is so important.

You do not fill your car with the quantity of petrol you are told by some arbitrary authority on cars in general that it should need to cover a set distance. You determine for yourself, depending on the type of car you own, how much it needs for the given distance. Just as some cars can burn up petrol faster than others, so some people use up vitamins, minerals and other nutrients faster than do other people.

There is another problem. The whole idea of what is the normal requirement rests on the concept of 'the average human being'. There is no such thing as the average person for whom the average result is desirable. We are unique individuals. Some people, for instance, need 222mg of calcium a day, whereas others need 1,018 mg – nearly a five-fold difference. Roger Williams, a noted biochemist who did much of the early research on B vitamins in the 1930s, reported on this several decades ago, yet we still pay insufficient attention to biochemical individuality.[31]

There is another flaw in rigidly following the 'normal requirements' and it relates to what is health. Health is not simply the absence of overt disease. It is a state of total, physical, mental and emotional well-being. This state was recognised in the official definition of nutrient deficiencies although it is rarely referred to or acknowledged as such. The RDI, or Recommended Daily Intake, official figures, commonly used in Australia, America and Canada, are based more on the levels that will prevent overt disease (2 above) plus a margin (which hopes to reach 3 above) than on the levels that ensure total physical, mental and emotional well-being (4 above). The RDA or Recommended Dietary Allowance is more commonly used in the UK and is similar, with minor variations.

That is a broad overview of some of the fundamental considerations; now let's get down to the details.

As with the previous predisposing factors, you can have too little or too much, although in the case of vitamins having an excess is rarely a problem, but see below.

What Do Vitamins Do?

Nearly all the reactions, in every part of your body and in every compartment within your cells, are able to work efficiently when they are assisted or facilitated by a catalyst. Without the catalyst being present the reactions would occur very slowly, possibly at a thousandth of the normal rate, or less, or so slowly that they would be virtually at a standstill. These biological catalysts are called enzymes and are made of protein. The proteins are produced within your cells, under the direction of your DNA from the nucleus of your cell when it, in turn, is instructed to set in motion the procedure for manufacturing that specific protein by the message that comes in via the cell membrane from elsewhere in your body. These enzymes are powerful and are vital for the actions to occur appropriately. Yet a majority of them cannot produce the desired results on their own. They, in their turn, need helpers.

These helpers are known as coenzymes. Whereas the enzymes are made within your cells, the coenzymes come from outside. Almost all coenzymes are either vitamins or minerals. You cannot make them. They have to be delivered from your diet. This is why it is so important that you get sufficient of these nutrients from your food. A small amount of the coenzymes can help the reaction to occur slightly more efficiently, a plentiful supply of the coenzymes can ensure that the reactions run with the maximum efficiency that is possible, within your own genetic capacity. Because coenzymes are facilitators and not drivers, they rarely push a reaction to go further than is appropriate, as decided by the messages within your cells and the actions of your genes.

Not all vitamins act as coenzymes all the time, some of them have additional roles to play. In general the phytonutrients also have additional roles to play. Some may be antioxidants; some may be protective in other ways. The subject is vast and belongs properly in a book devoted to nutrition. What is relevant here is that you realise the absolute importance of having a generous and fully adequate supply of all the vitamins and that your diet should also contain generous amounts of all the phytonutrients that the various vegetables can supply. Just getting the bare minimum of the 'absolutely essential for life' substances is not sufficient for robust good health, to avoid cancer or to help you to overcome cancer or prevent a recurrence.

The Best Sources of Vitamins

For the above reason I have a strong preference, where possible (and it is becoming increasingly possible), for recommending food-source supplements of vitamins and minerals. They may not contain quite as much of each vitamin (as listed on the label) as a synthetic vitamin supplement, but all the other plant ingredients generally provide huge additional benefits in themselves and often improve the absorption, transport and utilisation of the vitamins and minerals themselves.

Even with the best possible diet, when you live in a city and buy food that has been transported, stored and possibly processed, it is virtually impossible to get all the nutrients you need from a diet of commercially prepared foods, even if the foods are organically grown. There is little doubt that the nutrient quantity of today's commercial foods is less than it used to be. Even organic crops can be grown on mineral-depleted soil, and almost all crops are harvested before they are fully ripe and therefore before they have developed their full nutrient complement. Nutrient losses then occur during transport and storage. Thus, compared to our ancestors, we are getting a relatively depleted diet. In addition, it is probable that our requirements have risen significantly in the past few decades simply because we have to deal with so many more physiological and chemical challenges to our body, not least those caused by the toxins that surround us, the electromagnetic fields that are now a permanent part of our environment and the irresolvable stresses with which we live on a long-term basis.

The Effects of Low Vitamin Levels

A lack of adequate amounts of vitamins and phytonutrients is a predisposing factor for cancer for many reasons. In broad, sweeping terms it can weaken your immune system, leave your body vulnerable to damaging oxidation reactions, deprive your cells of oxygen and reduce your energy production. Anything that weakens your health in general leaves you vulnerable to developing further health problems. Knocking a rampart from one part of a castle wall may not lead to its defeat, but it is a significant step along the way and will lead to serious destruction if the process is repeated often enough; so it is with the human body. Vitamins are vital for the maintenance of good health and the prevention of diseases, including all the various degenerative diseases, up to and including cancer. If you have cancer you will need many of the vitamins in particularly generous amounts.

A few, more detailed, examples of deficiency-induced damage are:

The Krebs Cycle (a cyclical sequence of eight reactions, explained in Chapter 16) cannot operate without vitamins B_1, B_2, B_3, B_5 and biotin, and without that cycle your correct aerobic conversion of foods into energy is compromised. When the function of the Krebs Cycle is compromised, healthy aerobic-dominant mitochondrial metabolism is inhibited and the cell's metabolism becomes dominantly that of the anaerobic pathways that should, in a healthy cell, be playing a lesser role in energy production. This means that cells can all too readily revert to primitive (anaerobic) cancer-type metabolism. You will learn more about this in Chapter 16.

A deficiency of vitamin B_6 will inhibit your protein and amino acid metabolism. B_6 is an essential coenzyme in almost all reactions involving amino acids. If these are compromised, you cannot build up the protein you need for structure and function. You cannot make the various peptide hormones your body needs or the proteins that are required by your immune system, and you cannot make adequate amounts of all the enzymes (remember, all of them are proteins) needed for the thousands of different reactions that go on (mainly, but not only) inside your cells. Compromised enzyme production assuredly leads to compromised health, be it the health of your immune, endocrine, digestive, respiratory, genito-urinary, reproductive, cardiovascular, muscular-skeletal system, or any other part of your body.

Without sufficient vitamin C the adrenalin and noradrenalin that you need to deal with the stresses, good and bad, of daily life, are turned from the beneficial hormones to their toxic forms, adrenochrome and noradrenochrome respectively. Your immune system will be compromised; your white blood cells are the most vitamin-C-hungry cells in your body and they both need and store large amounts of it. Without vitamin C they cannot properly do their job of protecting you.

A lack of vitamin C in sufficient quantity can cause scurvy. This is a disorder in which your connective tissues break down, and it leads, as the early sailors found, to teeth falling out and pains in all the joints, tendons, ligaments and muscles, and more. This connective tissue includes compounds such as collagen and elastin. These in turn are made, dominantly, of three amino acids: glycine, lysine and proline. The lysine and proline, in a reaction catalysed by vitamin C, are modified so that they can form cross-linking bridges between the thousands of individual protein strands and hold the whole connective tissue together. Without vitamin C your connective tissues fall apart. Without vitamin C the ground substance, in which your cells sit, is weakened. When this ground substance is weakened, any roaming cancer cells can more readily penetrate, establish a new home and grow into a metastatic tumour.

Antioxidants protect your tissues from carcinogens.[32] Without adequate quantities of the antioxidant vitamins, such as vitamins A, C, and E, Phase Two of the cancer process can start unhindered and proceed apace. Vitamin C is vital in the fight against cancer.[33]

Vitamin D$_3$ has been shown to be one of the most important vitamins in the fight against cancer, and at levels considerably higher than the usual recommended intake. Countless studies show that it is difficult to overcome cancer if you are deficient in this vitamin, which is intimately related with calcium and magnesium metabolism;[34] however, an excess of this vitamin can also cause problems and, if you are taking large doses of 1,000 IU or more you should have your level checked every few months.

A lack of almost any vitamin can weaken your immune system and reduce your ability to prevent or overcome cancer.

I have already indicated that nutrient requirements are unique to the individual. If you blindly follow the recommended amounts, as provided by a range of text books on nutrition you may still not be getting sufficient for your own individual needs; however, at least that is a start. After that, you can do tests to find out your own levels either directly, by measuring the amounts in your blood, or indirectly, by assessing deficiency signs. There are several ways of doing this, listed below, but we will start with the basics.

Testing for the Vital Signs

There are several tests that can be done for vitamins. The first one you can do yourself.

1. Keep a diet diary

Although this can be time-consuming, a diet diary is one way to check your vitamin levels; you can do it yourself and it costs nothing. Write down all the foods you eat, daily, for a week, including the amount of each food. Then refer to a reference guide, with the nutrient content of each food, available at the back of many books on nutrition (particularly those that are text books), or go to the web for help.[35] Note the amount of each nutrient in the individual foods. This is best done on a spreadsheet with columns for each nutrient. Then add up your daily intakes for each nutrient and note the total. This is a tedious process, but it can be done. At the very least the amounts should match or be greater than the Recommended Dietary Allowance.

The recommended daily amounts of nutrients

It is no simple matter to establish how much of each nutrient you require for your unique metabolism and activities. To give you a flavour of the complexity, here are a few of the basic details.

- Daily Reference Values or DRVs are generally used for macronutrients.
- Recommended Dietary Allowances or RDAs, were developed in 1941 by the US Food and Nutrition Board who revised them every five to ten years. These are generally used on most UK supplements.
- Dietary Reference Intakes or DRIs were introduced in 1999 and based on recommendations from the Institute of Medicine (IOM) of the US National Academy of Sciences.

These DRIs are composed of:

- Estimated Average Requirements or EARs, which are levels that should provide sufficient for about half the population, the 50 per cent that require less than the average amount.
- Recommended Dietary Allowances or RDA, the daily dietary intake level of a nutrient considered sufficient to meet the requirements of nearly all (97–98 per cent) healthy individuals in each life-stage and gender group. It is approximately 20 per cent higher than the EAR. Note the words 'healthy individuals'. If you are not *totally* healthy, you will almost certainly need more.
- Adequate Intake, or AI, used for nutrients for which there is no established RDA, but the amount indicated is generally thought to be adequate, possibly with a less secure foundation.
- Tolerable upper intake levels or ULs, give an indication of safe upper levels.

The RDA is used to determine the Recommended Daily Value (RDV) which is printed on food labels. Note that it is the amount that is sufficient 'for nearly all' (but maybe not you) healthy people. But how healthy are you? Do you already have all your nutrient needs? Is this to be a maintenance level or the amount you need as part of your Optimising Strategy or health-improvement programme? These uncertainties are why you are advised to do some of the various tests in the Chapters 10–12. The RDA levels are rarely enough to restore health if you have any health problem at all. Remember that even the US Food and Nutrition Board, mentioned above, recognised, and stated, that total health was not defined as the absence of overt disease, but as a state of total, physical, mental and emotional well-being.

Daily Reference Values for the macronutrients are as follows:

Total fat	65g
Saturated fatty acids	20g
Cholesterol	300mg
Sodium	2,400mg
Potassium	4,700mg
Total carbohydrate	300g
Fibre	25g
Protein	50g

Assuming an average caloric intake requirement of 2,000 calories, the Reference Daily Intakes for several of the vitamins and minerals are as follows:

Nutrient	RDI	Highest RDA or DRI
Vitamin A	3,000 IU	10,000 IU
Vitamin C	60 mg	90mg
Thiamin, B_1	1.5mg	1.2mg
Riboflavin, B_2	1.7mg	1.3mg
Niacin, B_3	20mg	16mg

Nutrient	RDI	Highest RDA or DRI
Pantothenic acid, B_5	10mg	5mg
Pyridoxine, B_6	2mg	1.7mg
Folic acid, B_9	400µg	400µg
Cyanocobalamine, B_{12}	6µg	2.4µg
Biotin	300µg	30µg
Vitamin D	400 IU	600 IU
Vitamin E	30 IU	15mg (33 IU if synthetic)
Vitamin K	80µg	120µg
Calcium, Ca	1000mg	1300mg
Magnesium, mg	400mg	420mg
Iron, Fe	18mg	18mg
Chloride	3,400mg	2,300mg
Chromium	120µg	35µg
Copper	2mg	900µg
Iodine	150µg	150µg
Manganese	2mg	2.3mg
Molybdenum	75µg	45µg
Selenium	70µg	55µg
Zinc	15mg	11mg

Which nutrients are you deficient in?

Ensuring that your diet and supplement programme are providing you with at least the RDA levels of all the essential nutrients is a first step. Discovering any individual deficiencies can be helpful in indicating gross deficiencies in your diet. It can be a useful starting point and can provide clear insights as to just what you are doing to yourself by consuming your current diet; however, there are a couple of problems that this method does not address.

Firstly, remember that not all tomatoes are created equal and some will have more of each nutrient than others. This is true of vitamins, as the various vitamins are manufactured within and by the plant. The amount the plants make will depend on the way they were grown, harvested, transported, stored and, finally, treated in your own home.

Secondly, this method does not take into account your own unique requirements. For these reasons it is better to determine either the level of all the essential nutrients within your body and/or whether or not nutrient deficiencies are indicated by other parameters. Do the tests.

2. Determine your blood vitamin levels

A second method for determining your vitamin status is to analyse a blood sample for the levels of the individual vitamins; however, this only gives you the level of each vitamin in your blood at the moment the blood sample was drawn. This can be a useful general guide, but it will not necessarily give you an overall perspective on your total levels over the long term. In addition, some vitamins are not easy to determine in this way and the cost of laboratory testing is high. In general, this is not the most useful information to get. The information is included here for completeness.

3. The basic blood biochemistry test

This test is commonly carried out by your doctor and includes tests for vitamins B_9 (folic acid) and B_{12}. This information could help you if you are fatigued, as a deficiency of either of these vitamins can lead to anaemia. This test is not, and is not intended to be, a test for nutrient levels, other than for B_9, B_{12} and one or two minerals; however, if the results of this test are subjected to a computerised analysis, it is possible to learn about other possible deficiencies and to derive other useful information. Even if your results from this test are all within the 'normal' range, your health will be very different if some of the items are close to the top of the normal range, or close to the bottom of the normal range, or if one is near the top and another one is near the bottom, than if they are all centrally placed. This computerised analysis of the results from the blood test is done by Dr Patricia Kane of Body Bio and can be organised through Nutri-Link.

Why does your doctor not analyse the results in this way? This is a frequently asked question. The answer is that the information mostly focuses around nutritional or lifestyle issues and your doctor is almost certainly not well versed in these, certainly not to the level that we are considering here. If your doctor does not know how to handle the answer, he or she will rarely ask the question.

4. There are many indirect tests for deficiencies

These tests do not measure the absolute amount of vitamins in your blood. Instead, they assess the way your body is functioning, mostly at the cellular level. Many of these functions rely on a range of vitamins. This means that if a particular function is inadequate then functionally you are deficient in at least some of the necessary nutrients. This is generally much more useful than simply knowing the absolute amount of each nutrient that is present in a particular part of your body, such as the blood, or a body secretion, such as urine, saliva or sweat. You don't measure the efficiency of your water supply by measuring the amount in the tank, you measure it by what actually comes out of the taps and is available for use. The Optimal Nutrition Evaluation test or ONE test is one such example. Full details are on page 95.

There are several other tests that indicate nutrient deficiencies as bi-products of the main topic of investigation but they are complex and should be discussed with and organised by your CAM practitioner.

Your Optimising Strategy

Vitamin deficiencies are serious predisposing factors for cancer. You cannot protect your body from carcinogens or restore your body to better health if you are vitamin deficient.

The first treatment step is to boost your vitamin intake by way of your diet. Look for foods that are particularly rich in the missing nutrients as indicated by the tests you have done. In general, vegetables will often be indicated, but this is not always true and you should refer to nutrient tables in books on nutrition to find the best sources. Make sure that you choose nutrient-dense foods; that is, those that give you a lot of the desired nutrient in relation to the number of calories they supply. One of my earliest books focused on this,[36] there may be other more recent ones but I am not aware of them.

You will almost certainly need to take supplements of the vitamins in which you are deficient. If you have done the ONE test your report will indicate which vitamins are needed. So the second step is to take supplements that supply the missing vitamins. You should take these at least until your repeat test results show a total absence of any functional vitamin deficiencies. In all probability you will also need to keep taking them at some level to remain fully supplied; after all, the good results were based on the time when you were taking them. You don't eat only once, when you are hungry, and then expect to remain satisfied forever. Eating is an ongoing requirement, and the same is true of ensuring an adequate intake of essential nutrients such as vitamins and the minerals I discuss in the next chapter.

Vitamin deficiencies are dangerous. It is impossible to say which vitamin is the most important, just as it is impossible to state which is the most important link in any chain; however, a lack of adequate amounts of such important vitamins as vitamin A and the various carotenes, vitamin C, vitamin D_3, vitamin E (preferably as succinate) and the vitamin K complex can contribute to the cancer process and are certainly required if you are trying to reverse out of Phase Two. Remember, testing for vitamin D_3 is particularly important, as very high levels are often indicated and can be highly beneficial if you have cancer, yet an excess can be toxic. A simple blood test for vitamin D_3 can guide you and many laboratories offer this test.

The simplest solution to an anticipated vitamin deficiency is to take a good-quality multivitamin; however, you will need to read the labels carefully to ensure you have the full range and generous quantities. The cheaper supplements are unlikely to give you all you need, and by doing the appropriate tests you can better target your supplement(s) to suit your needs.

That was the vitamins. The other half of the essential micronutrients is the mineral group, which I discuss in the next chapter.

CHAPTER 12

Predisposing Factor No. 4 – Mineral Deficiencies

Just as you need a range of vitamins for good health, it is important that your body receives a range of minerals, both the macro-minerals, such as calcium and magnesium, and the micro or trace elements, such as manganese and molybdenum. Mineral deficiencies can adversely affect almost all aspects of your metabolism and increase your risk of developing cancer.

Your body needs all the essential minerals, but perhaps the most important one, when you are concerned about cancer, is selenium.[37] This is closely followed by such antioxidant minerals as zinc[38] and manganese.[39] Any mineral deficiencies, but particularly these, can set you along the path towards the cancer process.

What Minerals Do

Minerals play many different roles in the body. Like the vitamins, they often act as coenzymes that assist the enzyme catalysts. Zinc and magnesium, for instance, are coenzymes for several hundred different reactions. Minerals can also play structural roles, such as the calcium and magnesium found in your bones, plus their associated trace minerals, such as zinc, strontium and boron. Minerals can perform other functions: zinc assists the action of insulin; chromium assists the cellular uptake of glucose; sodium and potassium are essential for the passage of messages along nerve cells; iodine (classed as a 'mineral' physiologically, although the true chemist will have a problem with this, thinking of it as a non-metal) is part of the thyroid hormones T3 and T4.

You cannot make minerals in your body. They must all, without exception, come from the foods you eat. There is also a major difference between vitamins and minerals that affects their levels in foods. Vitamins are made within and by the plants that you, or the animals, eat. All being well, all tomatoes produce, and so contain, vitamin C, all whole grains produce and contain several of the B-group vitamins, albeit in varying amounts. The plants make the vitamins and they do this for their own good, so that they can survive and function. Minerals, on the other hand, cannot be made within the plants; they have to come from the soil. If the soil on which a plant grows does not contain zinc there can be none in the plant. The plant's health may be compromised but it may still grow and look healthy, yet when you eat it you won't be getting the zinc you presume it contains.

Most agricultural practices add nutrients to the soil only if they are vital for the growth of that plant, not if they are important for your health. It is the aim of most horticulturists to grow the biggest and most financially rewarding vegetable, not the most nutritious one for you the consumer. This means that using food nutrient tables to determine mineral levels does not always give accurate results. There can be a wide range of trace element concentrations in specific foods if grown in different locations and on different soils.

As the years go by, more and more minerals are recognised as being essential. When I started in practice it was not thought that zinc was an essential mineral; now it is known to be vital for a large number of enzymes and is included in mineral supplements. Elements such as boron, vanadium and molybdenum were barely mentioned; now we know that these all make important contributions to our health and they too are included in many supplements. It is probable that in future we will come to recognise more minerals as having health benefits. Man-made mineral supplements today contain many more minerals than they did a few decades ago. Future supplements may contain even more, as we learn about them. This is another reason for choosing plant-derived supplements. In general, and if made from sources grown on mineral-rich substrates, they will contain many more minerals than the man-made supplements; they will contain whatever was in the soil and taken up by the plant from which the supplement was made. So they will contain the ones for which the product was tested, and which are on the label. They will also contain others, potentially beneficial ones, that were not tested for in the product and which we may not yet consider to be important, although in future we may come to realise that, indeed, they are.

Deficiencies of almost all minerals can impair your cellular metabolism in ways that can increase your risk of developing cancer. To avoid cancer, make sure you have all the minerals your body needs. If you have cancer then you will need to make good any deficiencies if you want to recover fully and stay in remission.

Testing for the Vital Signs

There are many different tests that can be done for minerals; all have some benefits and possibly some deficiencies.

1. Hair mineral analysis

A hair mineral analysis is a useful and relatively inexpensive test. Individual hairs are made up of chains of amino acids. Among them, in relatively high concentrations, are the amino acids cysteine and cystine. These contain sulphur and give rise to the hydrogen sulphide smell you may have noticed when hair is burned. The sulphur atom has a strong affinity for minerals, and the sulphur atoms the amino acids contain are sufficiently exposed that they can combine with minerals. As the hair forms, and before it grows away from the hair follicle, it is exposed to the minerals in the bloodstream, which it absorbs.

The first 2.5cm (1in) of hair growth, measured from the root, reflects the mineral content of your blood for the past four to six weeks. It should be collected in several small bunches from a number of places across the back of your head, cut as close to the skin surface as possible. In the laboratory it is then analysed for a range of essential minerals. Analytical Research Laboratories, Trace Elements, Doctors Data and others offer this test. They will post you sample kits, on request and provide useful and comprehensive reports of the results.

This analysis is more reliable for some minerals than for others and you are advised to have professional help in interpreting the results. Nonetheless, deficiencies of trace elements in your hair frequently mean that there is a deficiency both in your diet and in your tissues. Selenium, for instance, is a vital antioxidant mineral, important in a range of reactions that help protect you from cancer. In the Keshan Valley in China, 30 or more years ago, it was found, by analysing hair samples as well as other tissues, that there was a gross deficiency of selenium in the soil coincident with a high incidence of cancer and heart disease among the people.[40] When the selenium deficiency was rectified the incidence of cancer and heart disease decreased.

Toxic elements can be detected in hair sample as cysteine will readily combine with minerals such as aluminium, arsenic, cadmium, lead, mercury and excess copper. If these elements are detected, you should focus on removing them during your detox programmes (see Chapter 15). Chlorella is a useful detox agent, especially for mercury and cadmium toxicity.[41] The amount in your hair is probably only the tip of the iceberg.

There are obvious advantages when using hair as a sample medium. Hair samples are easily cut, stored and posted to the testing laboratory. Instructions as to where you should cut the sample will come with the sample kit you receive from the laboratory; the samples can readily be sent by post without special labelling or packaging and they do not deteriorate over time. The test is inexpensive in relation to the amount of information you receive. Keep in mind that if you want information about your recent minerals levels, you will need to take the first 2.5cm (1in) closest to your scalp. The tip of your hair, especially if it is very long, will represent mineral levels that were present many months, or even years, ago, and even these levels may gradually have altered with repeated washing and other hair treatments.

2. Blood samples

It is important to understand that some minerals, such as magnesium, are preferentially taken up by the red blood cells (and so this medium should be sampled) and others dominantly remain in the plasma (which should therefore also be tested). Your practitioner, or the laboratory you use will be able to give you advice on the way they recommend you test blood samples for the minerals that are of particular interest to you. Red blood cell analysis is generally a good method for both essential and toxic elements. It is particularly good for establishing levels of potassium, magnesium and selenium.

3. Urine analysis

Samples of urine are readily collected and are often tested. Genova Diagnostics and Biolab offer such tests, as do several other laboratories. The laboratory will send you a sampling and collection kit complete with instructions. You can do a 'non-challenge test' by collecting a standard urine sample, and this will be indicative of the amounts of the minerals circulating in your blood. You can also do a 'challenge test'. In this, a chelating agent is administered that combines with minerals in your tissues and pulls them out and into the bloodstream, and hence into the urine; however, this should only be done under the advice of, and with the help of, a practitioner, as there are certain disadvantages to doing this, as well as benefits.

4. Sweat sample testing

You can measure the levels of certain elements, such as zinc, in sweat samples. This test is offered by Biolab.

Your Optimising Strategy

Mineral deficiencies make up predisposing factor number 4. If deficiencies are indicated, take the appropriate measures to make up what is needed in the same way as you did for the vitamin deficiencies, firstly by improving your diet and then, if necessary, by supplementing with the minerals in which you are lacking. The amount of supplementation required will depend not only on the levels found in your hair, urine or other sample but also on the extent of the deficiency signs you show in the rest of your body. Correcting mineral deficiencies is more complex than correcting vitamin deficiencies, as there are so many specific interactions between individual minerals. For this reason you are advised, for optimal results, to have professional help for this.

Once you have improved your diet and taken the appropriate supplements for a few months you will be well advised to repeat the tests to ensure that there are no more deficiencies. If deficiencies remain, you will need to increase your intake and to improve your absorption (see Chapter 13). If your levels have improved, this is not an indication that you can stop taking supplements; you may need to keep taking them possibly at a slightly lower level, to maintain these good results.

We have now considered the first four predisposing factors, what you eat, the foods and the individual nutrients. The next step is to assess what you do with them. That is the role of your digestive system.

CHAPTER 13

Predisposing Factor No. 5 – Faults of Your Digestive System

The fifth predisposing factor includes a large number of possible problems. It relates to difficulties with the state of your digestive system, to poor digestion (the breakdown of food into absorbable parts), and to poor absorption of nutrients from your intestines into your bloodstream. It can be subdivided into several components. Some of them lead directly to cancer, others, by hindering absorption of essential nutrients and harbouring toxins, can lead to nutrient deficiencies. They include:

- Problems relating to the state of your mouth, teeth, gums and chewing.
- Stomach problems, including inflammation (gastritis) and *Helicobacter pylori* (a bacterium), both of which are related to stomach ulcers and an increased risk of developing stomach cancer.
- Liver problems that relate to digestion and lack of adequate flow of bile. (Liver problems relating to toxins will be dealt with in Chapter 14.)
- Pancreas insufficiency and lack of pancreatic digestive enzymes.
- Damaged intestinal lining, and so reduced production of certain digestive enzymes, and reduced absorption of nutrients.
- Colon problems including stasis, the reabsorption of toxins and constipation.

Once your diet has been corrected and you have started taking the appropriate supplements, as indicated by the tests you have done, the next step is to ensure that all these nutrients are being absorbed. Only in this way can they reach their target organs. The foods have to pass correctly through your digestive tract and be properly broken down. If pieces of carrot, for instance, pass straight through your digestive tract and show up in your stool, you will not have absorbed the carotenes they contain. In practice, of course, it would be good to pay attention to this chapter at the same time as the previous two; however, we can only discuss them one at a time.

The Importance of Good Digestion

Much of the effort of obtaining a good diet can be lost if you do not digest your food properly. If you do not break the foods down into their component parts, into the separate fats, proteins and carbohydrates, and then break these down further into their individual fatty acids, amino acids and glucose molecules, then these valuable nutrients can be lost to you. It is essential that you release the individual vitamins, minerals and other phyto-, or plant, nutrients from their place within the foods you eat, otherwise you will not be able to absorb these essential substances. Instead, they will be passed out of your body, in your stool, without ever having been absorbed across your intestinal wall and into your bloodstream. If you do not absorb them they may even do harm on the way out, as they are then available to feed and nourish toxic organisms in your lower intestines.

Good digestion at a glance

You need to ensure that the conditions within your digestive tract are optimum for several reasons:

- To breakdown (digest) the food you eat so that it is available for absorption.
- To achieve efficient nutrient absorption.
- To maintain the correct internal environment within your digestive tract.
- To encourage the presence of beneficial organisms that will then produce vitamins and other nutrients for you to absorb.

- To inhibit toxic organisms that can themselves do direct harm, such as to your intestinal lining, and which can also produce toxins that can do harm both to your digestive tract and after they have been absorbed into your bloodstream.
- To eliminate waste material that has come (a) from your diet; and (b) from your body via your liver.

If your digestion is less than perfect the faults will flow like a row of spaced dominoes. The first one falls and the effect is felt all the way along the line. The end product, once the final domino has collapsed, can be a range of health problems that manifest anywhere in your body, up to and including cancer. If, for instance, you fail to absorb the fatty acids, you will have unhealthy cell membranes that may fail to respond to thyroid hormones, which will leave you with little or no energy.

You may feel that a small amount of indigestion is something you can live with – but you can't, it could herald much more serious problems either currently or building for the future. Do not be content to take an antacid and feel you can ignore the possible cause. I have had a patient whose doctor had diagnosed her 'heartburn' as 'indigestion' when in fact she had stomach cancer, and another who felt sure their problem was food poisoning when it turned out to be pancreatic cancer. Covering up problems of your digestive system with a quick pill is the worst way to treat them. It doesn't solve the problem and as often as not it interferes further with digestion. Passing wind is not something to feel embarrassed by and then ignore. It indicates a problem that should be nipped in the bud. Passing wind is not normal or healthy, even though it has become so commonplace that we tend to think it is.

The mouth

Proper digestion starts in your mouth, which can be the beginning of this predisposing factor. There are many requirements to be met here. They include:

- The production of sufficient saliva to 'hold' food together as you swallow.
- The production of enzymes – amylases – in the saliva that help you to break down starches.
- The production of an alkaline solution to maximise the action of these enzymes.
- A state of relaxation so that these fluids can flow. They won't if you are stressed or uptight.
- Time for the appropriate reactions to occur. It's important to chew your food thoroughly: 20 times or more for each mouthful.
- Healthy teeth and gums to ensure thorough and energetic chewing,
- Dentures, if worn, that fit correctly and comfortably for chewing salads, nuts and other raw foods.

The stomach

The next contributor to this predisposing factor is poor digestion in your stomach. For proper digestion to occur in your stomach, you need:

- Sufficient hydrochloric acid production to create the very low pH, or highly acidic state (discussed in Chapter 9), needed for breaking down the structure of the proteins you have eaten.
- Adequate output of digestive enzymes in the stomach – mostly, but not all, proteases or protein denaturing enzymes. These are enzymes that break down the structure of, for instance, a piece of meat, without breaking down the individual protein molecules.
- A healthy stomach lining so that ulcers do not form.
- The absence of bacteria that can harm your stomach.

The small intestine

Next come possible problems in your small intestine, and there are many requirements to be met before proper function is accomplished here. It is important that you have:

- Adequate pancreatic output of alkaline solutions and minerals to neutralise the acid mix coming from your stomach.

- Sufficient pancreatic enzymes. These are the lipases, amylases and proteases, needed for the breakdown of fats, carbohydrates and proteins respectively, into their molecular components.

- Adequate flow of bile from your liver, via your gall bladder, to emulsify fats and thus facilitate their breakdown.

- Sufficient flow of bile to stimulate peristalsis (the muscular movement that propels the partially digested food plus fluids, along the rest of your intestines).

- Adequate output of disaccharide enzymes on the intestinal walls to break down double sugars (disaccharides) such as sucrose, maltose and lactose, into their single sugar components, such as glucose, fructose and galactose.

- Healthy intestinal walls and intact micro villi (filaments) to provide the vast surface area that is needed for efficient absorption of nutrients.

- Transport molecules within the lining of your intestines to carry nutrients across the intestinal wall from your gut lumen into your bloodstream.

- The presence of beneficial flora or organisms. Good and bad bacteria (and other organisms) live in your intestines. The good ones both produce vitamins and aid digestion, the bad ones generate toxins.

- The absence of toxic organisms that alter the local conditions, produce toxins and interfere with the beneficial flora and inhibit digestion.

- Active production of secretary immunoglobulins (sIgA) for appropriate immune defence along the entire lining of your intestines, small and large (an area that has been likened to a football pitch). The amount must be sufficient to prevent the absorption of pathogens or toxic substances. In fact, this immune activity can constitute as much as 80 per cent of your total immune action. Think of it as guarding the most exposed and most vulnerable threshold to your body.

- Appropriate nutrients to protect the lining of your intestine.

The colon

The final contributor to this predisposing factor is made up of a range of problems that can occur in your colon. For healthy colon function you need:

- Sufficient non-digestible carbohydrate (as discussed under Fibre in Chapter 9).
- To avoid fermentation or putrefaction along the length of your colon.
- Good peristaltic action to keep things moving along.
- Regular emptying, not just once a day or a few times a week but as often as you eat, usually three times a day.

Improving Your Digestion Through Diet

The modern diet has contributed to many of the problems that occur in the digestive system. The good news is that this means you can do a great deal to correct many of them by improving the quality and nature of your diet. By doing the tests I will recommend here and by understanding the significance of the results you get you will learn just what changes you should be making to solve any problem you may have. Retesting will enable you to monitor your progress.

We'll now start the journey through your digestive tract in detail. In each section you will find a discussion of the possible problem(s) you may experience, the tests you can do and suggestions for treatments of any faults you find.

Your Mouth, Teeth and Other Oral Signs

Most people pay too little attention to the health of their mouth when they have indigestion. Yet digestion starts here, this is the first area in the domino line. If you have a dental problem, fix it. If you have mercury fillings they should be removed and replaced with safer compounds. Mercury is a serious toxin causing a variety of symptoms and encouraging the mould *Candida albicans*.[42] If you have root canals you should be aware that they could be infected, even if there are no obvious symptoms. Asymptomatic root canal infections have been linked with an increased risk of cancer, heart disease and senility.[43] If you have cancer, many practitioners will advise you to remove all root canals, whether or not they seem to be infected. If you want to prevent cancer you would be wise to remove this potential contributing cause from your mouth.

Gum disease and bad breath are generally thought of as a bacterial problem involving the gums. It could also indicate insufficient pancreatic activity. This makes it a predisposing factor to the development of cancer, since these pancreatic enzymes are part of your ability to destroy cancer cells.[44] If cancer is present, dentist William Kelley (who cured his own 'terminal' cancer, lived another 40 years, and helped many hundreds of other people with their cancer) suggested that the presence of gum disease could indicate difficulty in treating the cancer and the need for extra-large amounts of pancreatic digestive enzymes to break down the tumour(s).

The state of your mouth can also give you information about the rest of your body. If you have problems with your teeth and jawbone it could suggest that you have deficiencies of calcium, vitamin D or vitamin K and the beginnings of osteoporosis. If your tongue is 'geographic' or fissured, rough around the edges, coloured or blotchy, if you have sores in your mouth or in the corners, you could be lacking several of the B-group vitamins. Bleeding gums could suggest a lack of vitamin C and several of the different bioflavonoids.

Testing for the Vital Signs

See your dentist and have a thorough check-up. Be sure that he or she fully understands the dangers of both mercury toxicity and root canals in relation to cancer. If they don't, show them the books referenced here. If they still feel that mercury and root canals are safe, change your dentist. Ask around for one that suits your needs. There are many who are now concerned about mercury, but far fewer have caught up with the serious dangers of root canal fillings.

1   Take a good look at your tongue in a mirror. Check its colour, texture and edges.

2 Prod your gums to see if there is any area of tenderness, indicating the possibility of an infection.

3 Check for bleeding; you could be short of vitamin C and bioflavonoids.

4 Consciously consider whether or not you have sore areas within your mouth or along your lips or if you avoid chewing on certain teeth or parts of your jaw line.

Your Optimising Strategy

• Be sure to clean your teeth thoroughly. Floss or brush between them regularly.

• See your dentist for regular check-ups.

• Correct any dental problems that are discovered. It may be expensive, but it could save your life.

• Make good any vitamin deficiencies indicated either by local oral cavity symptoms or by other tests.

Problems That Can Occur in Your Stomach

There are several potential problems in this area.

Hypochlorhydria, or inadequate production of stomach acid

Your stomach contains a very strong acid, hydrochloric acid. It is meant to be strong – it could readily digest the muscles of your stomach wall, but this is protected by a thick mucilaginous layer. This acid is essential to denature the proteins you eat from meat, fish, poultry or other sources. It increases the acidity (lowers the pH) of the stomach to a level where the stomach's protein-splitting enzymes (proteases) are at their most active and digestion is optimised.

Many people produce too little acid, a state known as hypochlorhydria. Very few people, if any, produce an excess. Therefore you should not be concerned about any possible (although highly unlikely) excess of stomach acid. A deficiency of stomach acid on the other hand is a predisposing factor with many domino effects, because it compromises your digestion, and hence your absorption of nutrients, all the way down your digestive tract.

Surprisingly, without the strong prompt of acid leaving your stomach and entering your duodenum, your pancreas is not triggered to produce sufficient alkali to balance this acid, increase the pH and create the correct environment for its own enzymes to work in the next section of your digestive system, the duodenum. It's the domino effect again. These errors lead to faulty digestion and possibly induced intestinal fermentation.

These can lead to localised gases and to pain, all of which are too often put down, incorrectly, to too much acid, simply because we know that acids can hurt.

Hypochlorhydria is relatively common and often goes unnoticed or unreported by the medical profession. When this occurs the acidity of your stomach contents does not become sufficiently high (or the pH does not fall sufficiently low), and as a result the stomach's proteases cannot work efficiently.

You need the acid for proper digestion, but you produce less when you are stressed because your fight-or-flight mechanism – your sympathetic nervous system or SNS (Chapter 9) – is then in operation and not your internal-housekeeping system – your parasympathetic nervous system or PSNS. If you are dealing with cancer, you are stressed, so it is particularly important that you make the effort to relax while you eat and let your digestive juices flow correctly,

Symptoms and tests

Pain If you are experiencing stomach pains (under your left rib cage) it is probably not because of a lack of stomach acid. The more likely cause is damage to, or ulceration of, your protective stomach lining. It will have become weakened, possibly as a result of stress, and particularly if you have been eating when stressed or on the run. Remember that when you are in the active, or SNS dominant mode (Chapter 9), your digestive processes slow down, and so there is less protection for your stomach lining. This is the beginning of an ulcer.

This explains why you should not simply take alkalis (antacids) to neutralise the stomach acid and so reduce the pain; you should repair the stomach lining and keep the precious acid that you need. Slippery elm powder, 1 teaspoon when pain occurs, can put a protective cover over the area, and aloe vera juice, sipped slowly, can encourage healing.

Wind If you experience bloating in the stomach, or the need to burp, you may also be deficient in stomach acid, as the gases can be the result of improper digestion of the proteins.

Test 1 The simplest test is to purchase a supplement containing hydro-chloric acid from a health-food shop and take one or two tablets with meals. If your digestion improves then you have both detected and solved the problem.

Test 2 A method that is readily available and that your practitioner may do in their office is the dark-field live blood analysis. If your practitioner does this test they will look at a drop of your blood under the appropri-ate type of microscope and look for certain telltale signs that generally correlate with hypochlorhydria.

Test 3 A method that is being trialled and is well worth exploring with your practitioner is as follows. A capsule, containing a heavy but inert substance and attached to the end of a piece of string is swallowed. The other end of the string is taped to the outside of your cheek. You will then be asked to lie on your left side, which allows the capsule to fall into your stomach. After seven minutes the capsule will have fallen off the string, and the string will have soaked up the liquids from where it is lying along the length of your oesophagus (food pipe) and within your stomach. The string is then drawn smoothly and swiftly out of your mouth, a reagent is rubbed along it that changes the colour of the string with the changing pH. If the string turns red or orange this indicates an acid pH and this should occur at the distal end of the string where it was lying in the stom-ach. If it turns dark green this is alkaline and this should only be found at the near end of the string at the top of the oesophagus, nearest to your mouth. This test is offered via NutriLink.

Test 4 Another test for stomach acid level that is indirect but claims to have some merit is the salivary epithelial growth factor (EGF) test. It is known that when there is a lot of stomach acid, increased amounts of EGF are produced to protect the mucous linings of the stomach and associated mucous membranes. It has therefore been hypothesised that in conditions of hypochlorhydria, the level of EGF would be low. Clinical results suggest that this could well be the case and the test could be worth doing if you want some evidence before taking in extra acid in supplement form. The test is offered by John McLaren Howard at Acumen (see Resources).

Test 5 A stool analysis will also give information about stomach acid.

Your optimising strategy

Your first option should be to stimulate your own production of stomach acid. How often have you heard people say, 'Relax before, during and after eating'? This is not just a rule for good manners. There is a fundamental reason for doing this. It is so that your sympathetic nervous system is turned off and, as a result, your parasympathetic nervous system can come fully into play. Remember, when you are challenged, tense, anxious, worried or irritable, your sympathetic nervous system will be operating. Your parasympathetic nervous system is then automatically turned off, its actions being inappropriate. It can only come on again when you relax.

So, for the proper flow of stomach acid, as well as other aspects of the function of your digestive system, follow the dictum: relax before, during and after you eat. If you don't you will experience a variety of problems within your digestive system. They may seem minor at the time, but they can initiate many much more serious problems in the years ahead.

In general, as people age, their output of stomach acid decreases, and so it may be appropriate and beneficial to take a supplement containing hydrochloric acid on an on-going basis, possibly one tablet with each meal, or with each large meal. If taking them makes your digestion feel better, you will know that that is what you needed.

To stimulate the further production of stomach acid, make sure you have sufficient amounts of all the B-group vitamins. Two tissue salts, Nat Mur and Kali Mur, both available from health-food shops, can also help.

Stomach ulcers

Another stomach problem that compromises the rest of your health and is therefore a predisposing factor is ulcers, mentioned briefly above. In the past, many stomach ulcers were attributed to stress; however, it is becoming increasingly apparent that many ulcers are either caused by or associated with *Helicobacter pylori*, an acidophilic or acid-loving bacteria. This is thought to be the only organism that can tolerate the extremely acidic conditions found in your stomach. These bacteria are helical in shape, hence their name, and they can use this shape to 'corkscrew' their way into the mucous lining of your stomach or duodenum, causing inflammation, weakening the lining so that acid can get through to your stomach or duodenal wall, and finally creating an ulcer and possibly, eventually, cancer. It is also possible that the bacteria can be there but not, as yet, causing symptoms. So initially they may go undetected.

Ulcers may not lead directly to cancer, but they do increase your risk of increasing other predisposing factors such as nutrient deficiencies and faults further down the digestive tract, which in turn are predisposing factors. The presence of *Helicobacter pylori* is known to be associated with increased risk of stomach cancer,[45] probably as a result of the induced chronic inflammation and the consequent cellular changes. If you test positive for this organism, you should certainly take action to eliminate it.

Testing for the Vital Signs

There is a simple self-test you can do for yourself, at home, if you think you have a stomach ulcer. For this you will need to have on hand some aloe vera juice and some pure slippery elm powder (available from health-food shops).

The moment that you experience the pain you associate with a possible ulcer, mix one teaspoon of the slippery elm powder into some food or liquid (a small amount of mashed banana is excellent, as it is similar in texture). Swallow this and sip a tablespoon of aloe vera juice. If you have an ulcer, the slippery elm powder will form a mucilaginous covering to your digestive tract, rather like applying an internal bandage, and the aloe vera will start the healing process. The pain should stop. If it does, then an ulcer or ulcerated area is what you have. These same two remedies can be used on an ongoing basis until bacteria, if present (see overleaf) is removed and the ulcer heals.

John U

I recall when John first came to see me he had frequently experienced such excruciating stomach pains that he had been submitting himself to the emergency ward of his local hospital several nights a month. They did their battery of tests but could find no cause for his problem and were considering some serious surgery. He did the above test for himself, found it helped enormously and then followed the protocol below for healing the ulcerated area and had no further problem.

If you have any sharp or burning pain over your stomach area, it is worth testing for *Helicobacter pylori.* You can do a simple breath test. The laboratory you choose (and many of them do this test) will send you a kit with instructions. You breathe into the tubes provided, seal them and return them. The laboratory then checks for evidence of compounds produced by the *Helicobacter pylori.*

The second test is a stool test where evidence of the bacteria is looked for in the stool sample. Again, instructions and a sample kit are sent to you by the laboratory and your practitioner can arrange this for you.

Treatment

If the bacteria has been found, further action is required.

1   Make sure you drink your full quota of water – this is important. Avoid soda, juice, milk, tea and coffee. Eat lots of fruit and vegetables, sufficient to achieve an alkaline-residue diet. Broccoli is particularly helpful.

2   Include in your diet the oils indicated in the diet section (Chapter 9) such as hemp, coconut or flaxseed oils. Coconut oil is made up of approximately 50 per cent lauric acid, a medium-chain fatty acid. Lauric acid is helpful in itself, but it has the added benefit in that some of it is changed into monolaurin, a monoglyceride that is anti-bacterial, anti-viral and anti-protozoal. It can destroy the lipid coating on viruses such as HIV, herpes simplex, cytomegalovirus and many influenza viruses,

helping to block their expression, and it is active against *Helicobacter pylori.*

3 Eat as much garlic as you can. Firstly, the anti-bacterial substance, allicin, in garlic disrupts the bacteria's ability to create and maintain its cell membrane. Secondly, it inhibits excessive activity of the cell's DNA and RNA and so inhibits the formation of further bacteria. Finally, it removes the -SH group (sulphur atom) from the cysteine amino acid, which is found in many enzymes that are important for the normal functioning of bacteria, viruses and protozoa. In all these ways it helps to stop or reverse the production and growth of the bacteria. You may be wondering why, if garlic is harmful to this bacteria, it does not also harm you. The reason is that your body (a) makes less use of the -SH group in this way and so is less reliant on it; and (b) is protected by antioxidants such as glutathione peroxidase. Glutathione peroxidase protects you from oxidative damage; it needs selenium as a coenzyme (hence the importance of selenium if you have cancer), so make sure you get sufficient of this trace element.

4 Colloidal silver acts against many bacteria including *Helicobacter pylori.* You can use it to wash fruit and vegetables and can also drink diluted amounts of it. Propolis tincture, available from health-food shops, can help; add a few drops (see the label on the bottle you buy) to water and drink this two or three times a day.

5 The presence of *Helicobacter pylori* in combination with a deficiency of vitamin C has been found to contribute to stomach cancer. Treatment with vitamin C has been shown to inhibit *H. pylori.* Treatment with 4g of vitamin C a day for four weeks has been shown to eradicate the bacterium by 30 per cent compared to patients who were not given the vitamin C.[46]

6 A number of other supplements can also help or may become necessary. For example, any stomach problem can reduce the production there of intrinsic factor, a compound which is needed to assist in the absorption of vitamin B_{12}. So if you have a stomach problem, a lack of stomach acid production, a stomach ulcer or any similar digestion problem, additional amounts of this vitamin may be needed to help prevent an induced

deficiency. Vitamin B_{12} is a very large molecule, absorbed with difficulty if intrinsic factor is in short supply, and your doctor may decide to give it to you by an intramuscular injection. You may be advised to have one a month until your levels are normal.

Problems that Can Occur in Your Small Intestine

A lot happens in your small intestine, and consequently a lot can go wrong. Almost any fault here constitutes a predisposing factor, as it can have a major knock-on effect on the rest of your health. This is the place for the final breakdown of the foods you have eaten, and this is where the major breakdown of fats, proteins and carbohydrates occurs. The first part of this digestion occurs in your duodenum, at the start of your small intestine. The acidic mixture, known as chyme, arriving here from your stomach stimulates your pancreas to secrete alkalis and many different digestive enzymes, as already mentioned. These pancreatic juices enter your common bile duct and then flow into your duodenum. This is the work of your exocrine (external) pancreas.

Your liver produces bile, which is then stored in your gall bladder. Each time you eat fat it triggers the release of bile, which also flows down the common bile duct and into your duodenum. This bile acts as an emulsifying agent, keeping the fat globules small and so presenting a large surface area to the lipases – the fat-splitting enzymes – coming from your pancreas.

Gut permeability or leaky gut

The lining of your digestive tract has three major roles to play, all of which are vital for you if you are to be doing all you can to overcome cancer. It needs to recognise and let in the good guys, recognise and keep out the bad guys and act as part of your immune system. In other words, it needs to work assiduously to allow for and facilitate the absorption of essential nutrients while at the same time making sure that no toxins or pathogens (toxic organisms) are absorbed. It must have just the correct level and type of permeability. These two tasks are somewhat opposed to each other and a delicate balance of gut permeability has to be maintained. If it is not, then problems of either malnutrition or toxicity, or both, can occur. The third role lies within the overall immune system. Gut IgA (also called secretary IgA or sIgA in some reports), produced here, is an active immune agent essential for your protection from the ravages of infectious agents.

Nutrients are absorbed in two ways. Approximately 15 per cent of absorption is done trans-cellularly, or through individual epithelial cells. The nutrient enters the cell from the intestinal lumen, crosses it and then leaves the cell over the membrane on the other side and enters the bloodstream. Eighty five per cent of absorption occurs para-cellularly, or by slipping through the junctions between the cells. These actions are made use of in the test for faulty gut permeability, or leaky gut syndrome described below.

Testing for the Vital Signs

The extent to which your gut lining is intact (and not leaky) can be assessed by analysing a urine sample. The kit is obtained from the laboratory that will run the test. You are asked to fast overnight and then to swallow capsules of two sugar alcohols, mannitol and lactulose, neither of which are broken down within your body. These are safe sugars that are not converted into glucose and so will not upset your blood glucose level or feed cancer cells. Mannitol is absorbed trans-cellularly and easily; lactulose is absorbed para-cellularly and poorly. You are asked to collect a urine sample six hours after ingestion of the two sugars. This is then sent to the testing laboratory where it is analysed to see how much of each sugar has made it through the wall of your small intestine into your bloodstream and so to the kidneys and into your urine. An increased level of lactulose, measured as an increased lactulose-to-mannitol ratio suggests a leaky gut, as more lactulose than usual has been able to slip through the (increased leaky) gaps between the cells. This test is offered by Genova Diagnostics.

Your optimising strategy

Several steps are required to treat problems relating to the small intestine. They involve mucosal repair and protection, correction of intestinal flora, and correction of resultant systemic problems such as nutrient deficiencies.

1   Treatment starts in your mouth. Chew your food very thoroughly; this stimulates the flow of saliva and the production of epidermal growth factor (EGF), the polypeptide that stimulates the growth of new epithelial tissues lining the gut.

2   Your diet should be high in protein, complex carbohydrates from legumes (peas, beans and pulses) and vegetables, and fibre. Jerusalem artichoke flour has excellent healing properties. Psyllium seeds, flaxseeds and oat bran are also beneficial. The fibre is converted by colonic bacteria into short-chain fatty acids such as acetic, butyric and propionic acids. These are the main energy source for the cells of your colon. Low levels of butyric acid are found in people with active ulcerative colitis and Crohn's disease. Fibre decreases the intestinal pH and encourages the growth of beneficial organisms.

3   Vitamins, such as vitamins A and the carotenes, B_5 and the B complex, C and E, and the minerals copper, manganese, magnesium, molybdenum, selenium and zinc are helpful. Other helpful compounds include glutamine, glutathione and NAG, quercetin, FOS, gamma oryzanol (from rice bran), gamma linolenic acid (GLA), lipoic acid and phosphatidyl choline (in lecithin). Helpful substances or herbs include, ginkgo biloba and green tea, aloe vera, cat's claw, probiotics (beneficial micro-organisms), slippery elm powder (protective) and goldenseal (healing). They can be included in your diet or taken as supplements. You can try some of these on your own, but if the problem persists you should certainly consult with your practitioner.

4   Test for food allergens as discussed in Chapter 9 and avoid any allergens that are detected, as these can damage the intestinal lining.

5   Test for and treat any intestinal infestation or dysfunction. They both increase the damage to your intestinal lining and can contribute to a leaky gut. Prebiotics are substances that are not readily broken down in the digestive tract and that support the growth of the beneficial microorganisms needed for a healthy digestive system. They include oligosaccharides such as FOS (fructooligosaccharide), soluble fibre such as flaxseeds, psyllium hulls and slippery elm powder, and dietary fibre such as is found

in vegetables and whole-grain products. Probiotics are living microorganisms that are essential for good digestive health. They include lactic acid bacteria and bifidobacteria. Antiparasitics include caprylic acid and herbs such as garlic, wormwood or berberis. All three groups can help to restore a normal flora.

Problems That Can Occur in Your Colon

We have finally reached the last part of your digestive tract: your colon. This is often a badly treated part. This is where the residue of your diet lands up, prior to evacuation, but it is a long way from simply a holding area for waste products.

Your colon is where the relatively liquid waste is concentrated by the absorption of water back into the bloodstream. If this does not happen, your stool is watery and you have diarrhoea. If too much water is reabsorbed, your stool becomes too dry and is difficult to pass. This can happen if there is insufficient fibre in your colon to absorb and hold the water. The same can happen if there are insufficient beneficial bacteria in this area – often as a result of a lack of their food supply: the fibre you should have been eating.

We now know that absorption of substances through the walls of the colon into the bloodstream is possible. As a result some remedies can be given via this route. If your practitioner has advised you to have coffee enemas (explained in Chapter 15), this is where you can absorb the coffee which then goes directly to your liver to stimulate detoxification.

One of the major problems that can occur in the colon is constipation, a predisposing factor to cancer for the following reasons. Constipation leads to putrefaction and the production of many toxins that can cause both local problems and systemic problems as they are reabsorbed. As a result of the stasis all toxins are held in the area for far longer than they should be, increasing their potential to cause harm. In a constipated society it is no coincidence that colorectal cancer is so common and so lethal. It is the third most common type of cancer measured by mortality figures (lung, prostate, colorectal in men; lung, breast, colorectal in women), although it is the second most common by type in women after breast.[47]

Constipation – you may be surprised

How many bowel motions do you think you should have in a day? The answer may surprise you. One a day, or one on most days, which usually translates to about three to five times a week, is not enough. You should go as often as you eat. For most people this should mean going three times a day. Think about it logically. If you only go once a day then the waste material from the two previous meals has to sit around in your colon waiting for the third meal's waste to come down before the lot is expelled. In this time toxins, either already present or locally generated by fermentation and putrefaction can be reabsorbed back into the bloodstream from your colon. This is not desirable and leads to a toxic system.

Testing for the Vital Signs

The tests for constipation are simple, but they may not all be obvious to you. Several of them you can do for yourself.

1   Keep a diary and note how often you do pass a bowel motion. This is very much more helpful than relying on memory and wishful thinking.

2   You can look at the irises of your eyes. If there is a yellow or brown ring around the central pupil, you are constipated and there is a build up of toxins in the colon. This is true, no matter how frequently you have a bowel motion; after all, it may not be complete each time and there may be pockets of waste matter that remain left behind. This test is simple if your eyes are blue, green or grey. If your eyes are brown the discolouration is less clear but can usually be detected by careful examination.

3   You can measure gut transport time by eating an identifiable food that is unlikely to be totally digested. Dried corn kernels are excellent for this purpose. All foods should be digested, but it is common to find that such foods as corn kernels, or seeds such as sunflower seeds that have not been chewed, have survived the transit of your gut. You can also do the test by eating beetroot, once, and then waiting. Its bright red colour pigments will show up in the toilet bowl. Food should take between 24 and 40 hours, at most, to travel through your digestive system.

4   The Urinary Indican Test is a laboratory test undertaken by several of the listed laboratories. It may seem strange to analyse urine for bowel and digestive problems, but it reflects the fact that compounds can be absorbed from your colon. Many faults, such as an incorrect level of acidity, an excess of harmful bacteria or slow transit and localised fermentation, can lead to the formation of toxic substances in your colon that are absorbed back into your bloodstream. From there they go to your kidneys and are excreted in your urine.

Your optimising strategy

Start by correcting the basic fault and increase the amount of fibre in your diet. This almost certainly means increasing the amount of vegetables you eat. Remember, vegetable fibre is a lot more effective than whole grain fibre, although the latter is also helpful.

Make sure you drink your allotted amount of water, approximately 1 litre (1¾ pints) for every 22kg (50lb) of body weight, or 1.2 litres (2 pints) for every 22.5kg (60lb), of body weight. This water is then available for your stool and reduces the risk of it becoming small, compacted and hard, and therefore not stimulating peristalsis and being more difficult to propel along.

Do more exercise. By toning up your muscles, including your abdominal muscles, you can stimulate peristalsis.

Fibre supplements can help. If all this does not initially achieve the desired result, and it may not, as you probably have a lot of correcting to do, consider taking high-fibre supplements such as psyllium husks, flaxseeds (linseeds) or slippery elm powder. These non-digestible carbohydrates feed the colon bacteria, add bulk to the stool and hold water in it, keeping it bulky and soft. The increased bulk provides additional pressure on the colon wall and this helps to increase peristalsis.

Avoid the use of laxatives such as cascara or senna. Neither of these herbs correct the fundamental problem, the cause of your constipation. Instead, they irritate your bowel walls, cause a reactive evacuation, and leave your colon muscles no healthier or more active than before. These herbs are a prop rather than a solution.

If you cannot improve your bowel frequency you should seek professional help.

An unhealthy stool

A healthy stool was described at the start of this chapter. If there are faults, this is a predisposing factor for many reasons as discussed below; however, in addition to direct problems, the nature of your stool can provide other useful information.

Testing for the Vital Signs

You can test your overall digestive efficiency by observing this end product: your stool. You can do this yourself and you can also send a sample off to a laboratory for a more detailed assessment.

Examine your stool for its nature, and for undigested food particles, mucous, blood and consistency.

- If there is undigested food in your stool you need to improve the efficiency of your digestion. You may need to chew your meals more thoroughly, relax more while eating, take supplements of hydrochloric acid or pancreatic digestive enzymes or increase your fibre intake.
- Its consistency should be 'mushy' but just formed. It should not be in the form of hard lumps or hard pellets, nor should it be an unformed liquid. Something akin to the softness of cream cheese would be suitable. If it is either too soft or too hard you should increase the fibre content of your diet, preferably vegetable fibre.
- Some sources will tell you it should be large, somewhat like a small cucumber, but if you are having three movements a day, each one will obviously be smaller.
- It should neither sink to the bottom of the pan, nor form a slimy floater that is difficult to flush down the pan; the formed stool should float slightly.
- If there is obvious blood present, consider whether or not it could be due to haemorrhoids, or splits or cracks in your anus. The darker it is the more likely it is that the blood has come from some internal source and you should have this investigated by a professional.
- The presence of mucus suggests a variety of problems and you should also have this investigated.

It is worth emphasising, whether you are attempting to deal with health problems with medical drugs, CAM therapies or a combination of the two, that your digestive system remains your dominant delivery route. This cannot be said too often. You need a perfectly working digestive system if you want your foods to be broken down appropriately and to release their essential components so that these can then be absorbed into or through your intestinal wall and delivered into your bloodstream. Conversely, you do not want to consume or create and absorb toxins. You also need optimal absorption of whatever supplements or remedies you take.

For all these reasons, tests that help you to evaluate the state of your digestive system, that give indications for what improvements are needed and that can be used to monitor your success in correcting any errors, constitute a very important part of monitoring your health. Correct digestion and absorption are essential if you wish to avoid or overcome cancer.

To put this topic in perspective, official figures indicate that an estimated four to five million people in the UK suffer from identifiable conditions of the digestive tract, such as acute indigestion, abdominal pain and bowel problems. In fact the figure is probably a great deal higher. Many cases go unreported, others go unrecognised. As many as 90 per cent of the people in the country, possibly more, are probably constipated in that they fail to have three, soft, easily passed bowel motions a day. An American study covering only a three-month period found that in over 70 per cent of households someone had digestive problems sufficient for them to be reported. Problems with the digestive system are thought to kill 200,000 Americans every year. UK figures are probably proportionately similar.

Parasites and Pathogens

Before we leave the discussion of your digestive tract, we should consider what lives there and what impact those inhabitants have on your health.

To get the nomenclature right, pathogens are 'things' that generate pathologies or, in other words, cause disease, and many of them cause or contribute towards cancer, or hinder your recovery from cancer. They are usually living organisms such as bacteria or moulds. They may be viruses which hover between being living things and complex chemicals. The term can also be used to cover chemical toxins, although this is less common. Parasites are creatures that live on a host, in this case you, on which they rely for food, drink and shelter.

Some parasites will like the neutral conditions in your mouth. *Helicobacter pylori,* as you will recall, likes the acid conditions of your stomach. Other organisms may prefer the conditions of your duodenum, colon or elsewhere. Some will be floating freely and move through with the digesting food. Others will latch on to the inner surfaces and make a stable home for themselves and their offspring.

The bacteria

Your intestinal tract is not simply a hollow tube where food is received. It is a thriving metropolis teeming with life. There are more bacteria in your mouth alone than there are people on this planet, according to Sigmund Socransky, associate clinical professor of periodontology at Harvard.[48]

In full health the great majority of your bacteria are either beneficial or, at the least, not harmful. You could certainly not live without them. Many of them produce vitamins for you such as vitamin K, biotin and many of the B-group vitamins. Some assist in the process of digestion, some in detoxification, others help stimulate your immune system. Many are neutral, having found a comfortable home for themselves but not being inclined to help you in any particular way; however, they do help to take up space and so crowd out some of the pathogens.

Some of the beneficial organisms live in your colon where they feed on what is left of your meal after you have absorbed what you can. They get what you might consider to be the crumbs – the undigested fibre from your meals – so spare a thought for these guys and eat more fibre so that they get a decent meal. The organisms themselves can make up as much as 50 per cent of your stool, and so they need constant replacement by reproduction. They are needed for the bulk they provide you with and the moisture their presence helps to maintain in your stool, keeping it mushy and preventing constipation.

Unwelcome guests

The undesirable organisms or pathogens derive benefit from inhabiting your digestive tract, and then, unkindly, repay you by actually doing you harm. There are many organisms in this group, and whereas the beneficial organisms are generally small and often single celled, some of the pathogens can be quite large. Worms, for instance, can be many inches or more in length. I've had many clients who would have sworn they could not possibly have worms, who have done some enemas and have then been surprised to find lengthy worms either in their stool or even in the insertion tubing when it is removed and cleaned out.

A few of the parasites could, potentially, do you harm, but they are generally held in check by the existence and activities of the other two groups, the beneficial and neutral ones. Problems occur when this ideal scenario changes and the balance of the populations is upset.

A common pathogen, and a predisposing factor for cancer, that has achieved public notoriety is the mould, *Candida albicans*. It, like many of the other types, can damage the lining of your intestinal tract. When this occurs, several things happen. The damage it does to your intestinal walls can lead to a leaky gut, or increased gut permeability. This then means that toxins that were on their way out of your body in your stool, either those that came in during the previous meals (exogenous) or those that have been produced in your body and ushered out of your cells, blood or lymph and into your digestive tract, usually via your liver (endogenous), can sneak back into your bloodstream and recycle, thus continuing to cause you toxicity problems. Remember that, ironically, having a leaky gut can also mean that some of the valuable nutrients you want from your diet are not absorbed, another predisposing factor. An overgrowth of *C. albicans* can cause a lot of harm, locally and throughout your body. So can the presence of a wide range of other pathogens.

It is thought that we all have some of the mould in our digestive tracts from about six months of age, but that this is one of the pathogens that is normally kept in check by the presence of large numbers of beneficial bacteria; however, it can easily get out of control, particularly if you have used antibiotics or been given them during an operation. A large pro-portion of people with cancer, when tested, have been found to have an overgrowth of *Candida albicans* or a similar organism,[49] and it is impor-tant that this is detected (see below) and, if present, removed.

Testing for the Vital Signs

1 The bacterial overgrowth breath test

This test is based on the fact that many pathogens produce unwanted gases such as hydrogen and methane. A useful test involves collecting six samples of breath, collected at approximately 20 minute intervals, first thing in the morning, before eating or drinking. These breath samples are then analysed for the possible presence of unwanted gases, which indicate the presence of pathogens within your system.

2 The calprotectin test

Calprotectin is a calcium-binding protein that can kill unwanted bacteria and fungi, often as effectively as some antibiotics. It is produced by some of the white blood cells that are part of your immune system. High levels of calprotectin in your stool can indicate localised infections, damage to the intestinal lining, inflammatory bowel disease, the damage done by non-steroidal anti-inflammatory drugs (NSAIDS) such as aspirin, Chrohn's disease or the presence of colon cancer. Collecting a sample for testing is simple. All you need is a random stool sample, which is then sent, in the kit provided, to the laboratory for analysis.

3 Tests for *Candida albicans*

There are several tests that you can do for the presence of *Candida albicans*. The most common ones are carried out on saliva or blood, and because the fungi is so common and can cause such extensive symptoms, these are very important.

1   The first is a simple test you can do for yourself at home. This test should be done first thing in the morning before you brush your teeth. Spit into a glass of clear water. If you see any cloudy or stringy formation associated with your saliva it suggests that you have problems with fungi in general and particularly with *Candida albicans.*

2   There are formal laboratory tests you can have done for *C. albicans*, either on breath, blood or saliva. A saliva test can provide information as to the probable existence of a *Candida* overgrowth, and can indicate whether or not this overgrowth was in the past but is not now a current problem, whether it has only recently become a problem, or both. This information can help when a treatment plan is being formulated. A blood test is also possible and this is particularly useful if you are having blood drawn for another test, as it just means filling another tube.

3   If you are already planning to have a stool sample tested, it can also be tested for the presence of *C. albicans* and other moulds, the presence or absence of beneficial or pathogenic organisms and the presence of worms and similar large-scale parasites. You can also learn whether or not there is fermentation, the level of immunological activity, liver and bile function, the pH, the presence of undigested food particles or fibres, mucus, blood or undigested fats, and more, plus a full report with explanations.

    If you decide to do this full stool test you will receive, from the testing laboratory, a simple sampling kit and a hygienic container into which the sample is placed and enclosed and which is then posted back to the laboratory. In fact it is generally advisable to collect more than one sample, usually two or three, sequentially and at different times, and send these back together. The instructions will come with the kit. Genova Diagnostics offers this test.

When the results of some or all of these tests are taken together they can provide valuable information as to the overall state of your digestive system and other more subtle aspects of the way your body is functioning. They can then provide a rational basis for planning appropriate therapy and changes in your diet and lifestyle. They will also indicate whether or not further, more exploratory, investigation of your digestive tract is called for, and these tests can then be done sooner than might otherwise be the case.

Your Optimising Strategy

The treatment of problems related to parasites is an extensive subject. Many books have been written on the treatment of candidiasis[50] and these should be read for further details. In general, successful treatment requires professional help. However, there are things that you can do for yourself. Dietary changes involve the elimination of all sugars, as they feed many of the pathogens, and the reduction or elimination of all yeast-based foods. Some testing laboratories will also supply some suggested treatments.

You will need to boost the function of your immune system (see

Chapter 22), provide protection for your gut lining (discussed on page 144) and almost certainly employ a number of detox treatments, such as supporting the liver in its function and helping to clean out the intestines with coffee enemas (see Chapter 15). There are many herbs that can help to kill some of the pathogens, such as garlic, olive and oregano, but to accomplish this successfully it is important that you discover which pathogens are present.

The use of probiotics can then help to replace the pathogenic organisms with beneficial organisms.

Other treatments will depend on what the results show, and you should be guided in this by the health-care professional who has organised the test(s) for you; however, much of the information already given here may be applicable and could provide you with some useful ideas as you start to improve your digestive health.

Finally

This has been a lengthy chapter on your digestive system; however, it is a complex system and of fundamental importance to your health. It is vitally important that you correct any of the possible disturbances discussed here if you want to regain your health. Faulty digestion and some, or all, of its consequences are serious predisposing factors that can readily set you along the path of Phase One of the cancer process.

CHAPTER 14

Predisposing Factor No. 6 – Poor Liver Function

An organ that plays multiple roles in your life is your liver. It is intimately involved with your digestive system, and it is essential for eliminating toxins from the body. It could be argued that your liver does more jobs for you than any other organ; it is a lengthy and involved subject, but in this book we will be looking at it briefly.[51]

Digestion and Your Liver

We'll first take a look at the way your liver functions in relation to your digestion. Your liver makes bile. This is a complex fluid that contains bile acids, bile salts, cholesterol, lecithin and a range of other compounds, and it is essential for proper fat digestion. Bile is made continuously and stored in your gall bladder, situated on the underside of your liver, until it is needed.

Fats, such as those from your diet, do not mix readily with the aqueous fluids that flow through your digestive system. As a result of the mixing that goes on in your stomach, when the products of digestion first reach the duodenum the fat is in tiny droplets, but these, on their own, would quickly coalesce into large fatty globules. The fats have to be broken down by the lipases (fat-splitting enzymes) that flow from your pancreas into your duodenum, but when the lipases get there they can only act on the outer surface of each globule. For proper digestion to take place, therefore, and to help maintain the largest possible surface area for the lipases to attack, this coalescing of the fatty globules has to be prevented. For this you need an emulsifying agent. Bile is just such an agent. When you eat anything with fat in it your gall bladder is triggered and squirts some bile down into your duodenum for this purpose.

Your gall bladder

If you have had your gall bladder removed, not only is it probable that you will have some difficulty digesting fats but you also have an increased risk of developing cancer of the upper colon.[52] This is thought to be due to the continuous trickle of bile from the liver, bile that would have been stored in a gall bladder, if you still had one, and secreted only when needed.

Your liver acts on the foods you absorb

Nearly all the foods you eat go to your liver. It is your liver that processes the amino acids from protein and rearranges them so that those of which you have an excess are converted into ones that are in short supply. Your liver changes sugars, such as fructose and galactose, into glucose, the form in which your cells need and use it. Your liver is involved in converting vitamin D into its active form and in making the protein that transports vitamin A around your body. Your liver acts as a storehouse for B vitamins. The list is endless.[53]

Your liver plays a vital role in managing the fats and the cholesterol you eat. It changes what is commonly thought of as 'bad' cholesterol to 'good' cholesterol (from very low-density lipoproteins or VLDLs, through low-density lipoproteins or LDLs, to high-density lipoproteins or HDLs). Your liver is involved in the metabolism of your steroid and peptide hormones and of an enormous range of other compounds. Your liver is involved in your immune function.

In fact almost any problem with your liver can be considered to be a predisposing factor in that any such problem can have a serious knock-on effect all through your body.

Removing Toxins

Your liver plays a vital role in dealing with toxins, as we will see in Chapter 15. Removing toxins from your body is absolutely vital if you are to prevent or deal with the repercussions of cancer.

You have four routes for removing toxins from your body. You can eliminate them via your lungs (toxic volatile gases), via your skin and sebaceous glands, via your kidneys in urine and via your liver and colon in your stool. Of these four, your liver is by far the most important organ of detoxification, certainly when we consider the quantity of toxins it deals with.

Your liver has to deal directly with the toxins you take into your body as well as with those produced within your body: the waste products of your metabolism. When you look at the liver microscopically you can see rows of hepatocytes (liver cells) separated by sinusoids, or spaces. The structure is somewhat akin to that of a sieve. Your blood passes through this sieve and larger unwanted items, such as microorganisms and large metabolic waste products are removed. They are absorbed into immune system cells called Kupffer cells, which live within the sinusoids and whose job it is to break down the organisms and destroy their components.

After this physical separation, the chemical detox process in your liver comes into play. It is facilitated by a series of enzymes that collectively constitutes the P450 detoxification enzyme complex. This enzyme complex is responsible for Detox Phases One and Two (see below).

There are now thought to be three phases of detoxification plus the final elimination. For a successful outcome, all the phases must be operating efficiently. Failure to deal with toxins in this way is a serious predisposing factor to a range of degenerative diseases, including cancer.

Detox Phase One involves drawing the toxins out of your tissues. A large number of nutrients are required to accomplish this phase successfully. Some of these are antioxidants, such as proanthocyanidins, flavonoids, beta-carotene, catechins, and vitamins C and E. A number of minerals are directly involved, including copper, manganese and selenium. Other nutrients are involved less directly as coenzymes in related reactions. These include iron, magnesium, molybdenum, manganese and zinc, also at least three B vitamins: B_2, B_3 and B_6.

Detox Phase Two involves removing all this rubbish and collecting it up ready for disposal. Your liver becomes involved in a range of reactions that conjugate, or combine, various compounds with the toxins. In this way your liver prevents the mobilised toxins flowing around the rest of your body and doing additional harm, although it does mean you have a toxic and congested liver.

This phase also requires some vitamins and minerals, particularly vitamins B_5, B_6, B_9 and B_{12}, and the minerals selenium and magnesium. In addition, it requires a number of conjugating organic compounds. Many of these compounds are derived from or related to amino acids. They include acetate, N-acetyl-cysteine (NAC), glucuronic acid, glycine, glutathione, glutamate, methionine, sulphate and taurine.

This is perhaps a good time for you to stop and think back to earlier predisposing factors such as vitamin, mineral or amino acid deficiencies, referred to in previous chapters. You can now see how these deficiencies can compromise your liver's functions and render toxins particularly dangerous.

The activity of your thyroid gland is important in detoxification at this point. It has a direct effect on the P450 enzyme complex that is critically important for detoxification. A deficiency of the thyroid hormone T3 can decrease the level of certain of the P450 enzymes. So make sure your thyroid is functioning well (see Chapter 21).

Detox Phase Three is proposed by the medical profession, but not so well established, and is part of current research; however, it is of particular interest if you have had, or are considering having, chemotherapy for the treatment of cancer. This phase involves the active elimination of xenobiotics from the body. Xenobiotics are substances that are foreign to your body and that should not be there. They can be absorbed into your bloodstream from your digestive tract; they could also have come in via inhalation, injection or through your skin. It seems likely that Detox Phase Three ensures that any such xenobiotics that enter your bloodstream from oral intake are pumped straight back out, into your digestive tract, and so are rapidly eliminated. It is also thought to involve the pumping of xenobiotics out of your cells.

This process is obviously useful if the xenobiotics are unwanted or dangerous toxins; however, this mechanism can also apply to chemical drugs such as those used in chemotherapy and applied to cancer cells and this may be the reason why these drugs don't work as well as expected in some people who have a particularly active Detox Phase Three.[54]

The Elimination Phase is the final detox phase. It involves the elimination of the toxins from your body. This means making sure that there is good flow of bile from your liver to your gall bladder and from there to your small intestine. This accomplishes two things.

1   Firstly, the bile fluid will carry many of the conjugated toxins from your liver, especially those that are fat-soluble.

2   Secondly, as you will recall, the bile stimulates peristalsis and helps to prevent constipation, and so reduces the time during which these toxins could be reabsorbed back into your bloodstream.

This phase is assisted by calcium D-glucarate, which inhibits the intestinal bacterial production of beta-glucuronidase. Beta-glucuronidase, if present, would separate glucuronic acid, one of the conjugating agents, from the toxins with which it has combined in Phase Two. This would set the toxins free and available for reabsorption. Calcium D-glucarate can be obtained as a supplement if desired, but needs to be taken every four or five hours to ensure its constant presence in your small intestine.

Here is another reminder of the potential consequence of an earlier predisposing factor, in this case, constipation. Once again, increase the level of fibre in your diet. It is converted to butyric acid by the action of good bacteria, and the butyric acid in turn protects the cells of your intestinal walls. You can buy supplements of butyrate, but this does not remain in the digestive tract for long, and a much better solution is to ensure a steady production of butyrate by increasing your intake of plant fibre. Note that good bacteria have to be present, so if you have any pathogens, including *Candida albicans*, you should take probiotics, as already indicated, as well as the calcium glucarate.

The liver detox phases at a glance

Detox Phase One

Toxins are removed from the tissues using nutrients such as antioxidants (including vitamins and minerals).

Detox Phase Two

The toxins are collected ready for disposal by combining them with various conjugating organic compounds (such as acetate, N-acetyl-cysteine (NAC), glucuronic acid, glycine, and glutathione), with the help of vitamins and minerals. This stops the toxins from flowing around the body doing further harm; however, if they are not eliminated the liver becomes toxin laden.

Detox Phase Three

Xenobiotics (foreign substances) are eliminated from the body. Also eliminated may be chemotherapy drugs in people who have an active Detox Phase Three.

The Elimination Phase

Bile is used to carry toxins out of the liver and it also stimulates the speed at which they are removed from the intestinal tract as waste. Fibre and calcium D-glucarate can assist the process.

The Error of the 'Healing Crisis'

Many years ago, before these stages were fully understood, it was common to find people going on a water fast and accomplishing Detox Phase One but then getting headaches and feeling nauseous when Detox Phase Two didn't happen efficiently. Even today this can happen and is sometimes, and wrongly, still welcomed as a 'healing crisis' when in fact it is a strong indication that you are not supporting your liver and the activity of Detox Phase Two. At the very least, it suggests that Detox Phase One is happening faster than Detox Phase Two, and this should be avoided. You should either increase your intake of the supplements that support Detox Phase Two or slow down the activity of Detox Phase One by following more gentle (mobilisation) detox programme. This is obviously something you should discuss with your CAM practitioner but you will also find more details my book *The Liver Detox Plan*.

Similar symptoms are also possible if Detox Phases One and Two are happening faster than the final elimination. If this happens, there may be either a build up of toxins in the liver or in the colon with reabsorption of the toxins back into your bloodstream. Both can lead to nausea and headaches and to a general feeling of being congested, liverish or unwell. If these symptoms occur, you should, again, slow down your detox activities, especially Detox Phase One, and increase intestinal elimination in all the ways already described. I recommend that you seek advice as to how to manage your detox programme properly; after all, you do want to get rid of the toxins, you just need to do it safely. If you are having enemas (see Chapter 15), increasing their number will help to solve the problem.

Testing for the Vital Signs, and Your Optimising Strategy

We will assume here that you have ensured you have all the nutrients you need for Detox Phases One and Two. Specific requirements and possible deficiencies will have been highlighted by tests you have done for possible vitamin, mineral and amino acid deficiencies, such as the ONE test (see page 95). If you are not sure of your specific needs, take six capsules a day of my Liver Support, which is designed specifically for this purpose (see Resources).

Your liver is responsible for thousands of vital reactions. It will tolerate a lot of abuse, but in the meantime your health can gradually deteriorate. By looking after your liver you can help to prevent a range of health problems, including cancer.

CHAPTER 15

Predisposing Factor No. 7 – Toxins: The Silent Killers

The word, or concept of, 'toxins', as used in the context of this chapter, covers almost anything that harms your body. Toxins can be biological, chemical or physical, and so the term includes pathogens or toxic organisms, toxic chemicals such as heavy metals, toxic petrochemical products and toxic radiation and electromagnetic fields. To some practitioners the concept can also include emotions and toxic thoughts, but we will reserve that topic for Chapter 19.

Carcinogens are toxins, because they cause cancer, but not all toxins are recognised as direct carcinogens; however, even organisms or substances that are non-carcinogens but that are toxic to the body can constitute predisposing factors to cancer, as they interfere with the normal and healthy functioning of your body. A couple of examples will suffice. A toxin, such as mercury, that interferes with the Krebs cycle (explained in Chapter 16) can increase the possibility of the cell turning anaerobic and therefore cancerous.[55] The human papilloma virus (HPV) is closely associated with, and thought to cause, at least 99.7 per cent of cervical cancer and so could be considered a carcinogen as well as a toxin.[56] *Candida albicans*, on the other hand, is not directly associated with a particular type of cancer, but it is a toxin and does sufficient harm to many aspects of your metabolism that it can contribute to cancer, and so it too is a predisposing factor. Sodium benzoate is an allowed preservative found mainly in acidic food and drinks; on its own it is mildly harmful, but if it is used in a food or drink that contains ascorbic acid (vitamin C) then it is turned into benzoic acid which is a carcinogen and much more dangerous.[57] Similarly, the nitrates used to preserve meats and keep them looking bright red and fresh are moderate toxins, but when combined with amino acids (from the meat) in the acid environment of your stomach they are converted into nitrosamines, which are carcinogens.[58]

Toxins are a global, as well as a local and a personal phenomenon, and it is virtually impossible to live in this century and not be exposed to, and absorb, a large quantity of them. This is true no matter how good your diet or lifestyle; however, you can and should limit your exposure to them as much as possible. This is even more important if you have had, or are concerned about, cancer. I have not yet worked with a patient with cancer who has not had toxins in their body when tested. In fact, since the range of possible tests has increased to what is available today, I have not had a patient with any health problem who did not, when tested, discover that they had several toxins in their body.

Our Toxic World

We all live in a toxic world. There is overwhelming evidence for this statement. Toxic chemicals are added to our countryside by way of pesticides, insecticides, herbicides, fertilisers and a variety of other miscellaneous chemicals. It is conservatively estimated that 25 per cent of the population of Western countries suffer from heavy-metal toxicity[59] and that is only one small group of toxins. The *UK Pesticide Guide 2009* describes 1,300 pesticides alone, never mind all the other agricultural chemicals – and that is just a start. This should certainly make you decide to test your own level of toxic metals and toxic organic compounds. Arguably, the worst toxins are those that attach to your DNA and alter your genes, thus interfering with the way your cells function. Such an attachment can be the first, or an early, step in the cancer process. Tests for any of these toxins can, and should, be done.

Even if you do not do any tests for toxins it is worth going on a general detox programme, which is described later in this chapter. You may feel generally healthy, but you almost certainly carry a burden of toxins, and a good spring clean from time to time can be helpful.

Toxins we encounter every day

Thousands of different chemical toxins enter the food chain. They include those given to the animals whose flesh and produce you eat and those used to control plants and insects on the land. There are toxic organic compounds, many of which enter your body from your diet; including coloured dyes, preservatives, homogenisers, flavours, hormones, antibiotics and more.

There are toxins in your water supply and in the air you breathe. There are the many chemicals, a large number of them toxic, that can be found in cosmetics and lipsticks, skincare products, toiletries, toothpastes, hair treatment products and dyes, and perfumes. There are biological toxins such as viruses, bacteria, fungi and moulds.

Think about the chemicals you use in your home, the bleaches, polishes, detergents, oven cleaners, soap powders and removers, all topped off with dubious chemical deodorisers. In fact, although you may well complain of the pollution outdoors in the streets, the home is often a much more polluted place. Add to these the industrial chemicals, the street pollutants, the chemicals used in offices, factories and other workplaces, the petrol fumes in garages and the exhaust from cars, buses, lorries and aeroplanes. How can you be toxin-free?

Physical pollution includes wireless and the electrical fields and other energy disturbances from all the electrical equipment and wiring in your home or place of work, the surrounding buildings, offices, and so on. There is the bombardment of energies from mobile phones, from radio waves, television networks and more. There is concern, although the evidence is mixed, that these may be causing both physical and chemical problems, from oxidative damage in your body to neurological damage that could affect your immune and hormone systems and lead to the production of further toxic chemicals for your body to deal with.[60]

Just in case you are living in the country and feeling smug about your clean environment and your own organic home-grown vegetables, be warned. I have often found that such patients have many different toxins in their bodies, including those that have combined with their DNA and are thus capable of causing mutations. Agricultural chemicals can travel a long way and stay around for a long time. Even if you farm organically, it is unlikely that all your neighbours, or all the people from whom you live downwind, also do.

The (mythical!) average person eats up to 2kg (4½lb) or more of all these chemicals, combined, annually. If the chemicals were mixed and piled into a bowl, and you were told to eat the lot you would be horrified and would surely refuse. Yet you consume some of them every day of your life.

What the toxins do

An early step in developing cancer is often the attachment of toxins to your DNA, forming DNA adducts (or damaged DNA). These in turn can lead to genetic damage and mutations, and they constitute a serious predisposing factor that may be present and detectable long before there is overt evidence of cancer.[61] Their presence can serve as a warning that you should start a treatment protocol right away.

This is not a book about toxins – there are plenty of those; however, it is important that you realise how pervasive toxins are and how dangerous they can be. The presence and actions of toxins in your body, even if they are not direct carcinogens, are a serious predisposing factor. That is why the tests indicated below are so important. Carcinogens are, of course, an even more serious predisposing factor. (For further reading on this subject see Resources.)

Why Detox?

A regular detox programme is important for everyone, especially for people who are not perfectly healthy, and more so if you want to prevent cancer, or have or have had cancer. There are many reasons for this:

- You will be carrying the normal burden of toxins that are an inevitable part of life, almost anywhere on the planet and certainly if you live in an industrialised society.
- It is probable that any health problem you may have is, at least in part, due to additional toxins that you may be carrying.
- If you are sick, you will be producing toxins as part of the disease process. All inflammatory reactions, for instance, produce superactive and highly destructive substances called toxic free radicals.
- As you go about the business of improving your health, you will be releasing toxic matter, both from your own cells, tissues and body fluids and from any parasites or damaged tissues that you destroy.
- If you have had surgery, chemotherapy or radiation, your system will be laden with additional toxins including the anaesthetics, antibiotics and anti-emetics that commonly accompany surgery,

the chemo drugs themselves and the results of tissue damage following radiation and any other medications you have been given.

If you are going to reverse the disease process, it will help you enormously if you do the tests indicated below. This will be of benefit for several reasons:

- It will enable you or your therapist to determine what particular types of detox programme are necessary for you.
- You will know what toxins to look for, to source, and hence to avoid from then on.
- It will indicate what aspects of your metabolism are under threat and what nutrients you will need to support your metabolism until the detox is completed.
- You will be able to make the appropriate changes to your lifestyle so that you avoid or minimise any future intake of those toxins that are affecting you.
- It will help you to recognise what is happening if you have a detox crisis such as a flare-up of existing symptoms, or a burst of new symptoms, as you go through your detox procedure.
- You will, by repeat testing, be able to tell whether or not your detox programme is adequate. You may need to change or increase it until you achieve the desired result.

Testing for the Vital Signs

There are many different tests you can do. Some of them are specifically looking for toxins. Others have different purposes but also indicate the presence of toxins, often by their consequences on other aspects of your metabolism.

Toxic elements include minerals such as aluminium, antimony, arsenic, barium, beryllium, bismuth, cadmium, caesium, gadolinium, gallium, gold, germanium, lead, mercury, nickel, niobium, palladium, platinum, rubidium, silver, thallium, thorium, tin, titanium, tungsten and uranium.

Even some of the essential minerals can be toxic when present in excessive amounts. Copper, for instance, can be toxic and can cause hyperactivity, especially in children, if consumed in excess.[62] An excessive intake of iron can stimulate the activity of cancer cells.[63] Selenium, which is an extremely valuable nutrient – an antioxidant that is protective against heart disease and cancer – can also become toxic if consumed in excess. In fact, any mineral element, in excess, can cause problems and imbalances. Too little causes deficiency symptoms, the right amount causes benefits, and an excess causes overdose symptoms. There is a narrower window of benefit for the minerals than for the vitamins where the body can manage with, or benefit from, a very much wider range.

Home urine test for toxic elements

Some simple test kits for home use are available from Manifest Health (see Resources). They come complete with instructions and can be used to check a selected number of individual elements. The amount present is indicated by variations in colour once the urine test solution is mixed with the indicator solution. These are indicative only and high levels should be followed up by laboratory tests.

Hair analysis can detect toxic elements

You will already have read about hair analysis in relation to the nutrient minerals (pages 125–126). This test will also determine the levels of many of the toxic elements; however, the test will not detect toxic elements that are locked in the tissues and are not mobile. To mobilise and determine these you will need to use the chelating agents and urine test described below. Nonetheless, this hair analysis is a very useful starting test.

Urine analysis for toxic minerals

A generally useful test is based on a urine sample. A standard sample of urine, collected as described in the sample kit, can be collected at home and sent to the analysing laboratory. This will indicate what elements are moving around in your blood and being eliminated from the body each day.

If you want to know about toxic elements that are locked up in your tissues, you will need to do a challenge test to pull them out. This means taking a reagent such as EDTA, DMPS or DMSA. These compounds are chelating agents and as such they combine with any toxins in your tissues and pull them out so that they can be drawn into your bloodstream, from there they can be both detected on testing and eliminated in your urine. These chelating agents can be taken either orally or given intravenously. The chelating agents will also pull essential minerals from the tissues and possibly have other consequences, so it is essential that you talk with a qualified practitioner before you do these tests. Thus there are risks, but the urine samples taken following a reagent challenge give a much more comprehensive picture of your body's toxic load.

Blood analysis for toxic minerals

There are several possibilities with blood analysis. Whole blood can be analysed, the mineral content of the red blood cells can be analysed, as can the mineral content of the serum or plasma, the liquid outside the cells in the blood. Some elements occur in the serum or liquid of the blood, and others occur preferentially in the red blood cells. This has to be recognised when selecting the test medium, and your health-care practitioner who organises the blood draw should be able to advise you on this.

Sweat analysis for minerals

Tests for some minerals, such as zinc, give unreliable results when hair or blood is used as the sample. Zinc, and other minerals, can be tested for in sweat. Your practitioner will advise you on this.

Organic toxins

We have discussed toxic minerals. There are also literally thousands of toxic organic compounds in our environment, many of them derived from petrochemicals, and there are many different ways of testing for these.

You can test for pesticides and organophosphates, for petrochemical derivatives such as burned aviation kerosene, butane gas, natural gas, and diesel and petrol exhaust. You can test for food additives, for household chemicals, agricultural chemicals, for flame retardants, formaldehyde, p-dichlorobenzene and dimethyl phthalate. You can test for commonly used hair cosmetics and detergents and for volatile organic compounds. Obviously, this is a lot of testing and can become expensive. An alternative and efficient way to start is to do a single test for about 20 of the more common volatile compounds. Depending on what is found you can then decide what other tests might be needed.

Toxic DNA adducts

DNA adducts in your blood can be tested for. Acumen offers this test.

The Optimal Nutrition Evaluation

Among other components, the ONE test can highlight the possible presence of a number of toxins.

Neurotransmitters

In Chapter 18 we will be discussing neurotransmitters, the molecules that carry messages from and between your nerve cells. Some laboratories that test for neurotransmitter levels include tests for some neurotoxins, but check with the individual laboratory before committing to this test.

Your Optimising Strategy

If you have done some or all of the tests above you will know at least some of the toxins you need to remove from your body; however, it is impossible to test for all the thousands of compounds to which you are exposed, so it makes sense for you to assume there are many more. If you have not done the tests it would at least be reasonable to undertake a general detox, using some, if not all, of the methods detailed below. You can choose your own. From my experience with patients it is clear that some people are happy to fast and take Epsom salts but cannot contemplate doing an enema; others are happy to do enemas but would hate to have to fast. Other people take the matter more seriously and do them all.

Dietary-Detox Optimising Strategies

A simple dietary detox programme can take one of several forms. You can do the first two fasts any time you like, but many people who are working during the week report that Friday to Sunday, inclusive, is the best time.

A water fast and detox

If you are unsure about doing this, or you are diabetic or have an ongoing health problem that concerns you in relation to this detox, you should consult your practitioner, preferably one that understands the benefits of detoxing.

1   Do not eat for three days.
2   Drink approximately 1 litre (1¾ pints) for every 22kg (50lb) of body weight, or 1.2 litres (2 pints) for every 26.5kg (60lb), of body weight.
3   Support your liver with herbs such as milk thistle, dandelion and artichoke. As an initial guide, dosages will generally be indicated on whatever product you buy from your health-food shop.
4   Take the general supplement designed to support the liver mentioned on page 161.
5   On day four, have a day on vegetable juices and green salads, and then gradually return to a good, healthy diet.
6   If you have a 'healing crisis' with headaches, nausea, and so on, remember what was said on pages 160–161 and take what you need to increase the Detox Phase Two reactions and bowel eliminations.
7   Ideally, you should do this during a time when you can relax and pamper yourself. If you can't find such a time, do not use this as an excuse to avoid the detox. If you are working a regular week, start the detox a Friday and take it easy over the weekend. By Sunday evening your body chemistry will have adjusted to the lack of food intake, you will be operating on stored body fat rather than dietary carbohydrates, and you will probably feel a

lot better than you anticipate. The vegetables and juices on day four should be ample for that day. If you do feel unwell, this is a warning sign that there are problems to be solved and, again, consult your practitioner.

A juice fast

1   Follow the water fast above but use juices instead of water, using a similar quantity. The best juice fast would involve only green juices, made from a variety of green leaves, broccoli, celery, cucumber and herbs. Unfortunately, most people prefer carrot juice, which has a high sugar content. A small amount of this is acceptable, but the major component of the juices should be from green and other above-ground vegetables. Vary the combinations according to taste.

2   If you insist on a sweeter taste, use a combination of two parts carrot juice, one part celery juice and thee parts water. Add a small amount of ginger to the vegetables being juiced.

3   The juices should be made by you, at home, and drunk within 30 minutes of making them. Bought juices have been processed. When fresh juices are allowed to stand for any length of time the valuable components, such as enzymes and vitamins, gradually break down.

4   Remember that this is a detox programme. You should be aiming to both eliminate toxins and refrain from taking in any more, so of course all the vegetables should be organically grown and washed thoroughly.

Raw vegetable detox

Eat nothing but raw vegetables for a week with small amounts of steamed fish for protein and essential fatty acids. Protein is used up daily by your body. It is used for tissue repair and for making hormones, enzymes, neurotransmitters and other functional compounds. Your liver needs protein for its functions in general and, in the form of some of its amino acids, for the detox process. So it is wise to include some protein in any extended detox programme.

Fibre is essential

Remember that fibre does more than passively add bulk and prevent constipation, so consume generous amounts. If you have been exposed to any toxins, had surgery, taken any medical drugs, including but not limited to antibiotics and chemotherapy, ever had candidiasis, or experienced over-production of intestinal gas or bloating, you need to augment your beneficial bacteria as well. You will find several at your health-food shop. Some of the possible individuals are listed in the table below.

For the small intestine	Particularly useful for the colon. Can be taken orally or added to enema liquids
Bacillus subtilis	*Bifidobacterium adolescentis*
Lactobacillus bulgaricus	*Bifidobacterium bifidum*
Lactobacillus casei	*Bifidobacterium breve*
Lactobacillus fermentum	*Bifidobacterium lactis* (or *infantis*)
Lactobacillus paracasei	*Bifidobacterium longum*
Lactobacillus plantarum	*Lactobacillus acidophilus*
Lactobacillus rhamnosus	*Lactobacillus rhamnosus*
Lactobacillus salivarius	*Lactobacillus sporogenes*
Saccharomyces boulardii	
Streptococcus thermophilus	

So fibre and probiotics become an absolutely essential part of any programme be it for detox or against cancer.

If you make juices, do not throw away the valuable fibre. Pleasant fibres, such as carrot, ginger, fennel, and so on, can be used in a variety of recipes: to bulk up vegiburgers (preferably made by slow dehydration rather than fried) or as the basis for a delicious grain, sugar and fat-free carrot cake (just add ground nuts, spices and xylitol). An appropriate dehydrator and further information can be obtained from the Fresh Network (see Resources).

Specific element detoxes

Different toxins require different strategies for their removal, and so doing the various tests to discover what toxins you have absorbed will help you to plan a more targeted detox programme. For instance, black cumin can help if cadmium and lead are the problems, increasing your intake of molybdenum can lower an excessively high copper level, and chlorella can help you to get rid of mercury. Mercury is a particularly dangerous toxin in that it can cross the blood–brain barrier (BBB) and enter the brain where it can do enormous damage. Fortunately, zeolites, types of clay with a vast surface area and absorptive capacity, are available in supplement form, can also cross the BBB, and are able to absorb a large quantity of toxins in relation to their size and thus to draw mercury out of your brain. Taking chlorella in combination with generous amounts of fresh coriander (cilantro) can increase the detox power. The practitioner who organised the tests for you will be able to help plan the appropriate treatment protocol for you.

Targeted detoxes

Once you know which toxins are present you can find out the source, at least for some of them. If pesticides show up, you can assess your exposure to these. Perhaps detecting their presence will encourage you to buy only organically produced food. If there are toxic heavy metals present, or toxic plastic derivatives, again you can determine their likely source and limit your exposure to them. Parasites, if present, can betray themselves by some of the toxins they generate (they may also have shown up if you have had a stool analysis done). Knowing what the toxins are will help you to formulate an appropriate detox programme aimed at killing and eliminating these specific parasites.

It cannot be over-emphasised that it is important to learn what these toxins are and to consider where they could have come from, then to do all you can to eliminate these sources from your life.

Fortunately, there are many substances, phytonutrients, nutriceuticals and other agents, mostly plant derived, that can help in treating this problem, and you may also need to do some of the non-dietary detox treatments discussed below.

Although you can do much of this for yourself, it is essential to remember that you must not mobilise toxins from your tissues (Detox

Phase One) faster than your liver and other exit routes (kidneys, lungs and skin) can deal with them (Detox Phase Two – explained in Chapter 14), otherwise they can create further problems of auto intoxication. It is for this reason that I strongly advise you to consult your CAM health-care professional for guidance as to the best and most appropriate detox strategy for you. Toxins are dangerous and the danger varies with the toxin.

Non-Dietary Detox Optimising Strategies

As explained previously, there are four major routes of elimination: the skin, liver, kidneys and lungs. It is now time to consider these.

1 Skin

Detox via skin brushing Your skin can be considered to be the largest organ in your body. It has a large surface area compared to any other organ and it weighs around 2kg (4½lb), varying, of course, with your body size. Your skin cells absorb many of the toxins with which your skin comes into contact. These can include the chemicals in the various toiletries you apply to your skin, the cleaning agents, dust, dirt and grime picked up from inadvertent contact, as well as germs and other pathogens. Your skin can also take up toxins from the inside: from your bloodstream.

You lose a few billion of these skin cells daily in the normal course of events. Every time you brush against something, touch something or run your hand over your skin, dead cells fall away. These cells, in all probability, contain some of the toxins that are lodged in your tissues, They take these toxins with them as they fall, so regular skin brushing is an easy, free and convenient way to start your detox programme through this organ.

Use a sponge, loofah, or rough cloth, and give your skin a good work over in the shower or bath, or after some of the sweating detoxes described below. In addition to removing toxins and surface dead cells, brushing stimulates the fine capillary circulation to the outer layers of your skin and this in turn increases their uptake of whatever toxins were in your bloodstream. These will be eliminated when it is the turn of these cells to be brushed off.

Detox via sweating using hot baths, hyperthermia and foot baths
There are many other ways to encourage toxins to leave your body
through your skin. One of these is to induce sweating. You sweat continuously, whether or not you are aware of it. This occurs as part of your
normal temperature regulation. You start to sweat overtly at 37°C
(98.6°F). As your skin temperature increases, the amount of sweat
increases steadily. If you are of average body weight, and are moderately
active, you will lose up to 500ml (18fl oz) of sweat a day. You will be
unaware of this level of sweat production, called 'insensible perspira-
tion'. Replacing this lost fluid is one of the reasons you should drink
plenty of water daily.

If you apply heat, in the form of hot baths or a sauna, your output of
sweat increases as your body tries to restore its normal temperature.
Sweat can carry with it a number of toxins, including heavy metals,
alcohol, nicotine and other organic compounds. Just smell your sweat
at the appropriate time if you are inclined to doubt this.

The enzymes that are involved in the reactions of your immune cells
function best at temperatures above the normal body temperature
of 36.9°C (98.4°F). This makes obvious sense when you think about it.
You do not want to overwork these enzymes, and hence your immune
system when your temperature is normal. When you have an infection
your body generates a fever in order to raise your temperature and trigger your immune system into increased activity. The greater the infection
the higher the fever, so if you ever do get a fever, work with it, don't kill it.
When you do not have a fever, you can stimulate your immune function
with a hot bath. A short period of increased body temperature, will give
a brief stimulus to your immune system, which in turn can help to
increase the detoxing process.

There is yet a further benefit of applying heat. Cancer cells do not like
heat. In general, people who 'get a temperature' following the least
infections are less likely to develop cancer than those who say, often
with misplaced pride, that they almost never 'get a temperature'.[64] Heat
stimulates your bone marrow and increases its production of white
blood cells. Heat also stimulates your thymus gland and its output of
natural killer (NK) cells, all of which increase the activity of your
immune system.

It has been found that at a body temperature of around 44°C
(111.2°F) cancer cells die.[65] The problem with this is that at that temperature you are likely to start having fits and to do harm to yourself as

well as to the cancer cells. For this reason the medical profession has largely ignored the benefits of heat in helping someone with cancer; however, it is not necessarily a case of all or nothing. There is a good chance that even some heat can act against cancer cells, if to a limited extent – but every little helps. The CAM profession does recognise the benefit of hyperthermia, particularly when it is localised, and so is less of a strain on the rest of the body. This is a technical treatment and should only be done with specialised equipment and under supervision. You will need to ask around for a suitable clinic near you that offers this treatment.[66]

Before you go to these lengths, there is a simple protocol you can manage at home. This form of detox is cheap – just the cost of the hot water – and it is simple; it can be done on your own at a time of your choosing. You will get the maximum benefit from this if you can get your body temperature up to 38–39°C (101–103°F) and this can be done in a hot bath. In practice you will probably not reach this temperature. If you decide to do this, start slowly and gradually increase both the temperature of your bath and the time you remain in it. If you do feel faint at any time, get out of the bath, lie down and drink more water before you try again. Do not do this if you have a heart problem or high blood pressure, and if you are concerned, consult your practitioner.

Before you start, drink at least 500ml (18fl oz) of water to replace in advance the fluid you will lose as sweat. Drink a mineral or electrolyte solution such as athletes drink after sports (but without the flavourings or sugar) to replace the essential minerals that you will also lose in the sweat. You can increase the detox process by taking several chlorella tablets and 1,000 mg of quercetin before the bath.

Run a bath that is as hot as you can bear it. Add 100g (3½oz) of bicarbonate of soda (sodium bicarbonate, or baking soda, not baking powder) to the bathwater if you want to reduce your level of toxic acids, or the same amount of Epsom salts if you want to loosen up your joints. If you like, warm some essential oils over a candle – just to make the experience as enjoyable as possible. Have a good book to read, a glass of water to drink and a small towel to wipe off the sweat. Get in, lie back and enjoy for at least 30 minutes, topping up with more hot water as needed so as to ensure a continued sweat. If you are unsure about any of this, take advice from your CAM health-care professional.

You can further increase the benefit by wrapping yourself in a large towel as soon as you get out of the bath, going back to bed and piling the covers over you so that you continue to sweat for up to an hour.

Foot baths Large quantities of toxins can be drawn out of your body via your feet and their sweat glands. Foot baths are simple; all you need is a bucket deep enough to come well up your calves and wide enough to put both feet inside and flat on the base. Start with the water as hot as you can tolerate it. Have a kettle of boiling water beside you and keep adding this to the water your feet are in as it cools down. You can then add a variety of aromatic or detoxing herbs or herbal oils, or simply sit and either read or meditate for at least 20 minutes.

Foot bath and liver stimulant As above but add the following to the water: 1 teaspoon of cayenne pepper and 1 tablespoon of Dijon mustard (or less English mustard powder, but be careful not to blister your skin; start with ¼ teaspoon). Keep the water hot for the next 20 minutes by carefully topping it up from a hot kettle, making sure you pour in the water so that it does not touch your skin.

Fill a hot water bottle with near boiling water and wrap towels around it so that you can just place it over your liver, covering the lower part of your right rib cage. Hold it there for five minutes, then replace it with a cold pack (a bag of frozen peas will do very well) for another five minutes. Repeat the process a second time. This rapid change from cold to hot and back again helps to stimulate the flow of blood through your liver, and bile from your liver. Do this while your feet are in the mustard bath.

Foot bath with equipment If you put a search into the Internet for 'detox foot bath' you will find a number of suppliers of equipment designed to provide a more powerful detox process through your feet.

Far infrared detox saunas Infrared radiation is radiation with a shorter wavelength than that of the visible spectrum, beyond the red end of the spectrum. The wavelength ranges from 4 microns to 1,000. Far infrared (FIR) rays, as the name implies, are rays at wavelengths at the far (short) end of the infrared spectrum, furthest away from the visible radiation. FIR rays are the safest and the most beneficial rays that come from the sun.

Whereas infrared lamps give off a gentle heat and are often used in combination with, or alternating with, massage, FIR rays don't only act as a source of heat; they can penetrate 5–7.5cm (2–3in) into your tissues. They then gently increase your tissue temperature, increase the activity of many reactions and stimulate circulation. Finally, they stimulate excretion of toxins from your cells, which is then followed by their removal in the sweat induced by the rays. Some reports claim that the sweat induced by FIR is as much as 12 times more concentrated in toxins than the sweat induced by simple heat saunas.

For therapeutic purposes there are many types of equipment available that will generate and radiate high levels of FIR, usually between 4 and 14 microns, the wavelengths within which most body processes function and so which provide maximum therapeutic benefit (see Resources). One of the simplest available is similar to a duvet folded in half to make a sleeping bag, with Velcro along the bottom and up the side to close it once you are inside. Some FIR units are like half cylinders, cut lengthways, either solid or collapsible, under which you can lie and which have the FIR unit at the base. Others are like small box tents placed over a chair on which you can sit with just your head protruding through the top of the canvas. Finally, there are the entire FIR cabins, similar to a small sauna chamber. They all require electricity and they generate FIR that penetrates your body. The duvet or blanket, since it wraps so closely around you, is one of the best and also the most compact for storage.

Far infrared rays offer many benefits:

- They expand your tiny blood vessels, the capillaries, and so improve your circulation, increasing the flow of blood and the amount of oxygen available to your tissues. This increases the effectiveness of everything else that they do.
- They improve your fluid balance.[67]
- They increase your heart rate and output and thus further improve your circulation while also helping to reduce high blood pressure, if that is a problem.[68]
- They stimulate an increased loss of toxins from your blood into the sweat.[69]
- They activate your sweat glands and increase the loss of this fluid, together with the toxins it contains.

- They activate your sebaceous glands so that cosmetics and dirt that have accumulated within your pores are eliminated along with your sweat.[70]

- The action of many enzymes is stimulated by FIR rays, and so overall cellular metabolism is improved.

- The increased metabolism can lead to weight loss, if that is your aim, over and above the temporary fluid loss, provided that you don't eat to make good the calories you have lost in the process.

- At the same time FIR can help to break down cellulite, releasing further fats, toxins and water trapped in this tissue.

- Many parasites are killed by FIR.[71]

- FIR increases the production of white blood cells and NK cells, and so stimulates your immune system, which not only protects you from infections but also kills pathogens, thus removing their toxins.[72]

- In addition to all this detoxing, there is a constructive benefit from having an FIR sauna; it can stimulate the activity of fibroblasts, the cells that help to rebuild new tissue, and so help in tissue repair and wound healing.

- Further repair is accomplished by the positive action of FIR on DNA and protein synthesis so that new cells and tissue can more readily be produced to replace old and worn out or damaged cells. In this way it can further help to heal new wounds or old scars.

- FIR helps to balance the hormonal system.[73]

- FIR relieves nervous tension and relaxes tense muscles. This further assists in healing and helps to reduce pain, thereby helping the body make the most of its intended healing abilities.

- It can help to relieve insomnia.[74]

Even if you have not had cancer, you should consider having at least an hour's FIR sauna from time to time. If you have, or have had, cancer you could benefit from a daily sauna. A convenient-to-use sleeping bag-style FIR sauna is available from Get Fitt. A quick Internet search will locate others.

2 Liver and colon

Colon cleanse No matter how many bowel motions you have – and most people have too few – it is highly likely that you have impacted material in pockets in your colon. A colon cleanse will help to remove these. The first step is to dissolve 1 tablespoonful of Epsom salts in purified water and drink this first thing in the morning and then repeat this twice more at 30 minute intervals. This will give your colon a good clean out. Two hours later start drinking 500ml (18fl oz) of citrus punch (see box) every 30 minutes.

For a thorough cleanse, if you are constipated or are seriously ill, this process should be repeated for three consecutive days once every month.

Citrus punch

The punch is made from the juice and pulp of 12 oranges, 6 grapefruits and 6 lemons. These must be organic and you should wash the skins very thoroughly. Peel the fruits and reserve the peel. Blend the juice and pulp, then make up to 5 litres (8¾ pints) with purified water. If you like it sweeter, dissolve some xylitol in hot water and add it to the punch.

Do not waste the pith and peel, they contain even more nutrients than the pulp and juice – hence the reason for cleaning them thoroughly. The pith and peel can be dried in a dehydrator – at no more than 40.5°C (105°F) – and then ground to a fine powder. This powder can be added to salad dressings, desserts, Budwig mixes (see pages 101–2) or any other dish in which the citrus flavour would be appealing.

Enemas and your liver

We have already covered the way your liver deals with toxins and the supplements that can help to achieve this via Phases One to Three in Chapter 14. There are other ways you can help your liver to perform. The first is to do a coffee enema and the second is a liver flush.

Enemas are simple to do, painless, inexpensive and easy to perform, and are normally done on your own without help. In my experience most patients are reluctant to consider doing them when they are first advised to do so. Once they have done a few they soon become firm adherents to the practice, saying that the process and the feeling afterwards are things they would not like to forego. One previously reluctant client even announced that he would disobey me if I suggested he stop doing them. So put any preconceived ideas or concerns behind you and think about it as an enjoyable half hour to spend curled up with a good book.

Max Gerson was one of the early pioneers of the CAM approach to the treatment of cancer, advocating a diet of raw foods, vegetable juices and detoxing regimes. If you have read any books that involve CAM therapies for cancer, from the popular and well-known Gerson approach onwards, you will know that daily enemas are a necessary part of any CAM treatment for cancer, and arguably should be part of all treatments for cancer. This is true even if you have had the tumour removed surgically. It is even more true if you are breaking the tumour down with enzymes and other CAM treatments. You will have a lot of toxins to get rid of and daily enemas are essential, you may even need more, certainly at the start. Enemas are important to help you maintain a healthy body to support your liver and gall bladder,[75] remove toxins and prevent cancer or other serious degenerative diseases. Their importance was recognised by the medical profession until just over 30 years ago. They were described in the Merck Manual, the book of accepted orthodox medical treatments, from 1890 to 1977, when they were removed allegedly for lack of space, as new medical developments jostled for position. Coffee enemas were a regular part of the nursing arsenal throughout the early twentieth century.

Cleansing of the bowel goes back thousands of years, being described in many ancient medical texts. It is very common to find that the root of a person's health problems lies in the poor functioning of the bowels, and bowel cleanliness is essential for good health and well-being. But cleansing the bowel is not the only purpose of doing an enema. There are several others.

1   Clearing old and possibly long-term impacted waste from the colon. This is such an important topic that it is worth repeating that most people are constipated and you may be too.
    Compacted faecal material can putrefy in the bowel in pockets (diverticuli) for long periods, become inflamed (diverticulitis)

and produce toxins that are reabsorbed back into your bloodstream and so circulated around your body. This putrefaction also encourages the build up of painful 'wind' and of mucus inside the intestines, and prevents the efficient absorption of nutrients. It contributes to a decrease in the normal feeling of well-being and lays the foundation for many diseases. Some signs of a toxic colon can be headaches, skin problems, sore throats, fever and swollen lymph glands and that yellow ring around the central iris in your eyes mentioned on page 146.

2   During a fast it is especially beneficial to take enemas to improve the quality of the cleanse. During a major detox programme, or when breaking down unwanted tissues such as a tumour, it is essential, as the enema-induced elimination helps to prevent your body being overloaded by the mobilised toxins.

3   Enemas stimulate the colon wall, causing a reflex peristaltic activity in the remainder of the upper colon helping to restore normal function and healing. High enemas have been used even by people with colon cancer, but you should consult with your practitioner about this, if you are concerned. Their decision will depend on the location of the tumour within the colon and the degree to which it obstructs the colon or is vulnerable to abrasion. The concern may involve a tumour of the descending (left side) colon, the lower part of which is traversed by the enema tube. Remember, however, that any local tumour is exposed to the friction of passing faecal material and if you are even slightly constipated this will probably be rougher than the tube.

4   Coffee stimulates the liver to activate all the tiny channels within it, channels which may have become congested with toxins and bile. This frees up the liver to process more incoming toxic materials that have accumulated in the rest of your organs, tissues and bloodstream. Unlike coffee taken in by mouth, coffee absorbed in this way does not go into the systemic circulation (around the rest of your body), unless the enema procedure is done improperly or too much coffee is used.

5   Coffee contains choleretics – compounds that increases the flow of bile from your liver to your gall bladder and so to the intestines – where it improves fat digestion and stimulates peristaltic action, thus further increasing the movement of stool along your intestines and relieving constipation.

6   The coffee contains alkaloids that stimulate the production of glutathione-S-transferase, an enzyme used by your liver in the detox pathways. It is pivotal in the formation of more glutathione, one of the main conjugation chemicals that combines with toxins in Detox Phase Two and increases their elimination. In this way a coffee enema speeds up the detoxification process and minimises the backlog of toxins waiting to be eliminated.[76]

7   Coffee contains esters that are thought to stimulate Phase Two of detoxification and stimulate the liver to eliminate many times its normal amount of toxins.

8   Nutrients can be given via an enema. A typical example would be to add green tea to the enema solution and allow your body to absorb the beneficial catechins and other compounds in it. If you are doing an enema in the evening, shortly before going to bed, you may prefer to use green tea without coffee if the latter stimulates you too much, though this is, as said above, usually avoided by reducing the amount of coffee used. You can add yoghurt, or some powdered probiotics to the enema to add to the beneficial bowel flora, or chamomile for relaxation.

Doing the enema

There are basically two types of enemas: low enemas and high enemas. A low enema involves the insertion of a solid tube of only 2.5cm (1in) or 5cm (2in) in length. The main objective of this type of enema is to flush out the lower, or last part, of your colon, the rectum. If you are using the hard white tube insert it *slowly*, rotating the tube a little if you find this eases its insertion.

A high enema includes the use of a soft rubber tube, about 40cm (16in) long, that is added to the distal side of the enema tap and is gently inserted fully up your colon. Here the purpose is to maximise the absorption of some of the enema solution ingredients, such as coffee or green tea, to stimulate the liver for further detoxification and to give the colon a more thorough clean out. The most usual detox enema involves the use of coffee.

The last part of the colon, before reaching the rectum, is in an 'S' shape and called the sigmoid colon. By the time stool gets to this part of the colon, most nutrients have been absorbed back into the bloodstream. Have you ever felt sick just before having a bowel movement? It usually occurs when stool material has just moved into the rectum for elimination. The stool contains toxins and products of putrefaction and these may be being reabsorbed while they are waiting for evacuation. As soon as the material is evacuated and the toxins have been excreted, you no longer feel sick. The nausea was due to the toxic quality of the material. Because of this, it is important that you always evacuate when you have the urge. Do not hold on unless it is absolutely necessary. The rectum should usually be empty.

The procedure

The enema procedure is simple, it can be done easily at home, by you on your own, and the equipment is inexpensive. It is generally available from good chemists or via a health-care professional or Manifest Health (see Resources). It consists of an enema bag with a loop, so you can hang it from a hook or door handle. At the bottom of the bag there is a flexible clear tube with a tap at the far end. All this remains outside your body. The kit generally comes with a short rigid extension for insertion suitable for a low enema and this is attached below the tap. To this you can attach the long 40cm (16in) soft tubing if you plan to use that. The tubing to be inserted should be lubricated before use with aloe vera gel which is also healing, should this be needed.

The instructions will generally come with the kit or from the person that supplied you with the kit. In brief, while lying down, you allow the enema solution to flow into your colon. The solution should be made from medicinal, unroasted, organic coffee, using approximately 1 tablespoon in 1 litre (1¾ pints) of water. Then remove the tube, lie on your right side for 20 minutes or as long as you can hold it (this is where reading a good book comes into it), then sit on the toilet and let it go. A double enema means doing a second one 10 minutes or more after the first, and it is often possible to retain and absorb this one, which is then referred to as a retention enema. Adding a powdered probiotic such as *Bifidum bacterium* to this retention enema will help to inoculate the bowel with beneficial organisms. This can be especially helpful if you generally pass a lot of wind.

After doing an enema you will probably feel very much lighter and 'cleaner' than you did before. Most people enjoy this outcome. If you feel you are experiencing a coffee 'high' or getting the jitters, reduce the amount of coffee you are using. You should be relaxed after the enemas, and be able to do them before going to bed without disturbing your sleep. Always discontinue the enemas if there is any adverse reaction whatsoever, and discuss it with your CAM practitioner.

If you have an active tumour or are in any part of Phase Two of the cancer process you may want to do several enemas a day. If you don't have cancer but want to prevent it, it is wise to have one enema a day, as do some of my colleagues, but even if you do one a week it can be beneficial.

You may say that enemas are not natural and we should not need them. It is true, they are not natural. But then it is not natural to live in such a polluted world. It is not natural to be exposed to or consume all those toxins. We need a way of eliminating them. We use cars and other forms of transport (unnatural) instead of walking and running (natural). We live and work inside air-conditioned or enclosed buildings (unnatural) instead of being exposed to a ready supply of fresh air (natural). We stay up and are active for many hours after dark (unnatural) instead of sleeping when it is dark and rising at dawn (natural). We do many other unnatural things; enemas are just one more, and they counterbalance the unnatural toxins to which we are exposed. Remember that enemas were detailed in the Merck Manual until 1977.

Liver flush

The liver flush provides a stronger stimulus to the liver than is provided by enemas. It gives it a good work out. In brief, it involves first emptying out your digestive tract, then drinking sufficient olive oil to stimulate the maximum flow of bile, not only from where it is stored in the gall bladder but also from all the ducts within the liver. The bile is expelled from your liver and gall bladder, it then enters your small intestine and flows through to your colon, carrying with it all the stored toxins and, arguably, any small stones.

The procedure is relatively simple and is as follows, but before doing this you should follow a four-day work up to the process. During each of these days you drink, between meals, 1 litre (1¾ pints) of organically produced apple juice to which you have added 5g (⅙ oz) of orthophosphoric acid (which you can generally obtain from a chemist or health-food shop). Fresh apple juice is best, but bottled apple juice will do if it is of good quality. Rinse your mouth after drinking it to prevent the acid (from the phosphoric acid) damaging your teeth. If you suffer from candidiasis, or have been told to limit your sugar intake, substitute malic acid tablets (or magnesium malate) for the apple juice. During these four days eat normally and drink plenty of water.

On day five, eat breakfast and lunch as normal but take a tablet containing 1,000mg of calcium before each meal. Two hours after lunch (approximately four o'clock) take 1 tablespoon of Epsom salts dissolved in warm water. Add juice or xylitol, if you like, to mask the flavour. Take another tablespoon of Epsom salts two hours later (approximately six o'clock). The Epsom salts will trigger a major colon clean out. The worst part is now over and the next step is a pleasure. Two hours later (approximately eight o'clock) prepare a large bowl of fresh berries, whip up a generous serving of double cream and eat as much as you can, especially of the cream. This cream, (recommended by William Kelley, but it can be replaced by increasing the amount of olive oil used) has a serious purpose, namely to activate the liver and gall bladder. Take another 1,000mg of calcium. Do not eat anything else, but you can drink water.

Half an hour before going to bed drink a quarter cup of bentonite liquid, or drink one tablespoon of bentonite clay stirred into a glass of water. Then get undressed and completely ready for bed. Now comes the part that most people dread but is actually not nearly as bad as taking the Epsom salts. Drink half a cup of cold-pressed organic olive oil. Choose an oil with little or no flavour and try to imagine it is cream; after all, it feels much the same. If you think you will have a problem with this, have a glass of freshly squeezed grapefruit juice beside you and take a few sips.

Go straight to bed. Lie down immediately, on your right side with your knees drawn up to facilitate the oil reaching your gall bladder. Remain in this position for at least 30 minutes, preferably until you fall asleep. You may experience mild nausea; this is normal and will soon pass. If vomiting does occur there is no need to replace or top up the oil that is lost in this way.

You will probably wake during the night to evacuate your bowels. Have a fine mesh sieve handy. There will be almost no stool to pass but concretions or fatty 'blobs' are likely and you should collect these. They have little odour and are not unpleasant. These may be liver or gall stones, although this is debated. It is probable that some will be hard and others more 'rubbery'. First thing in the morning collect any more that come out. Count them. You can then monitor your improvement when you compare this to the number you collect on subsequent occasions.

When you wake on day six you will probably feel slightly tired and possibly slightly wrung out. It is best to rest as much as you can on this day. Eat lightly, preferably fresh salads, and gradually resume your normal diet. You will generally be back to normal by the evening and feeling a lot lighter and healthier than before.

Although this process is relatively straightforward, it is best to do it with the advice and supervision of your health-care professional, as it challenges the body more than an enema would. When my patients do one, I generally suggest that they tell me and time it such that they can phone me any time during the procedure, particularly during the night, if they have any questions or concerns.

If you have cancer, it is generally recommended that you do a liver flush once a month, no more. For prevention purposes and to improve your liver function, you could do one or two a year. A lot will depend on how good your diet is, how heavy your exposure to toxins is and on the state of your liver.

4 Kidneys

Your kidneys are at the head of another elimination route. They filter your blood and allow toxins to pass out into your urine while at the same time holding back beneficial blood components.

If your kidneys are sluggish, there are several things you can do. The first thing is to ensure that you drink plenty of pure water. The inappropriate use of strong chemical diuretics is not recommended; however, there are several herbs that have mild diuretic effects and also support your kidney function. One of these is dandelion. You can buy dandelion leaf tea, either loose or in tea bags. You can also buy the roasted root, marketed as a type of coffee. The roasted and ground root can be boiled, or an instant version is available in most health-food shops. Use these drinks to improve kidney clearance of toxins, but be sure to drink other fluids as well to replace an excessive diuretic loss. Your liver will also benefit.

5 Lungs

Your lungs are not part of a major excretory route in the way that your kidneys and liver are, but they do help to eliminate unwanted gases. Deep breathing will improve this and will also increase the amount of oxygen available to your blood and so to all of your tissues. Most people breathe only from the top of their lungs, taking short, shallow breaths. This may in part be the result of having been told in childhood to hold yourself straight and pull your 'tummy' in. Don't do this. At least don't hold your tummy in in such a way that you cannot drop your diaphragm and take deep breaths. Whenever you think of it, throughout the day, consciously take deep relaxing breaths in, and then slowly let them out as far as you can. Not only will this increase the exhalation of toxins but it will also draw in additional oxygen for circulation to your cells, and it will increase your state of relaxation and thus reduce your level of stress (see Chapter 19).

You may be getting rid of toxins by producing an increased amount of mucus via your nose, throat or lungs or an increased amount of ear wax. The latter is sometimes experienced following an operation. You may also be breathing in air that is loaded with dust or other particulate matter. An excess of mucus production may mean that you are allergic to some of the common foods; the most usual culprits are dairy products and wheat. The FACT test offered by Genova diagnostics can help you determine this.

Other ways to detox

There are several other ways to increase the elimination of toxins, but I have not discussed them here, because you will need professional advice for many of them. If you are interested in finding out more, I suggest you contact a CAM practitioner to discuss the methods that he or she can help you with. Lymphatic drainage can be helpful and there are several homoeopathic and herbal remedies that can assist. Colonics can also be helpful.

Although you may not feel prepared to do all or many of these detox procedures, they are all important and have their place in a thorough detox programme as Katie, opposite, discovered.

Katie R

Katie had had a tumour surgically removed and was encouraged – to the point, as she put it, of bullying – to have follow-up radiation. When she refused this she was warned that a recurrence was a near certainty and that it was highly unlikely she would be alive in two years' time. She refused the radiation and instead started on the programme described in this book. By her third visit she had determined her metabolic type, modified her diet accordingly and made sure that it consisted almost entirely of alkaline-residue foods. As a result, she ate a wide variety of vegetables (mainly raw), drank vegetable juices every day and derived her protein intake from yoghurt and flaxseed oil mixes with added whey protein isolate in powder form, plus small amounts of fish.

She did a variety of tests, gathered up the information on deficiencies and added the appropriate supplements and remedies to her diet. She was not, she said at this time, ready to start on enemas, buy FIR sauna equipment, or do a liver flush, but she did start on the other detox procedures.

Two months after her first visit, she was suddenly reminded to comment that her stiff joints had entirely loosened up, and she now found herself skipping up and down stairs instead of clinging on to the banister.

In the next few months, as she moved further through her programme, this improvement continued. She did eventually embark on a full detox regime, including enemas and liver flushes, and felt even better as a result. She had other tests for abnormalities and did what was necessary to correct the results. She held a celebratory party at the end of five years, to which her surgeon and would-be radiologist were invited (they did not come), and she remains in remission.

It is all too easy to underestimate the damage that can be done by even very small amounts of the many thousands of toxic chemicals in our present environment. These toxins can interfere with important metabolic processes, reduce the activity of vital enzymes and increase the risk of a range of diseases. Ideally, you should do the tests to find out which ones are compromising your health. At the very least, put yourself on some of the detox programmes described here.

CHAPTER 16

Predisposing Factor No. 8 — Fatigue and Faulty Energy Production

Fatigue in itself may not seem like a predisposing factor, but the fact that you are feeling it indicates the existence of a variety of underlying problems. There are two aspects to this predisposing factor.

The first part involves your body failing to produce all the energy needed by you and all your individual healthy cells. This can be due to a deficiency in the nutrients you need for cellular energy production and the resultant failure of the normal energy-producing pathways. Without the correct input or generation of energy, your cells cannot function correctly. When this happens your tissues cannot function correctly either. The cells of your liver, heart, lungs, muscles, pancreas, brain, kidneys, hormonal glands and all parts of your body need plenty of energy if they are to do their job properly.

The second part involves problems that arise when your cells start to revert to the method of generating energy that is indicative of more serious fundamental problems, and that is the method used when healthy cells turn into cancer cells.

Phase One of the cancer process, the topic for this book, is about prevention and does assume that you do not have cancer. But we cannot consider this aspect of cellular energy without considering the way cancer cells produce and use it.

How You Generate Energy

The first step is to understand how you normally generate energy at the cellular level in healthy cells. Energy comes from the combustion, in the presence of oxygen, of the carbohydrates and fats that you eat. The process is analogous to the combustion of wood in your fireplace to produce heat. If you have eaten more food than you need and there is an excess of energy available, the spare food-derived energy is converted into storage batteries, in the form of fat molecules that are stored in your adipose tissues.

First, we will look at how carbohydrates are converted into energy. One way or another carbohydrates almost all end up as glucose, which travels through your bloodstream and is, eventually, taken up by your cells. Inside the cells the glucose is broken down and its energy is released via two sequential pathways, the EM pathway and the Krebs cycle.

The EM Pathway

The first energy-producing pathway is the EM Pathway, which occurs in the oxygen-free, or anaerobic, cytosol or general matrix of the cell. Because this pathway occurs in the absence of oxygen, very little combustion of the glucose takes place, and very little energy is released; instead the glucose is reorganised. In this pathway each six-carbon glucose molecule is rearranged and finally broken down into two three-carbon molecules of pyruvic acid.

The next step is complex and pivotal. The pyruvic acid molecules in the anaerobic cytosol become acetyl groups, which finish up in the oxygen-rich mitochondria. The mitochondria are the organelles within the cell in which the majority of the energy is produced, approximately 90 per cent or more. It is thought that it is when mitochondrial energy production is compromised that healthy cells can turn into cancer cells.[77]

There are two possible outcomes, at this pivotal point:

1   The desirable one; and
2   The escape route if the desirable route is blocked.

There are many components to this pivotal and complex reaction and so, of course, there are many reasons why it can go wrong.

The pivotal-point reaction complex involves, and is dependent upon, the presence and the activity of a large number of vitamins and minerals. These trace nutrients include vitamins B_1, B_2, B_3, B_5, biotin, lipoic acid and magnesium. If you don't have enough of these nutrients in your diet you will have difficulty releasing the energy in your food, you will feel tired, your foods will not be broken down and will turn into body fat instead. You will also be pushing your cells from Phase One to Phase Two of the cancer process, as we shall see.

The Krebs Cycle

All being well, each acetyl group arrives in one of the many thousand mitochondria that exist inside each cell and the second pathway can start. This is an aerobic process and is a cyclical sequence of eight reactions called the Krebs cycle. In this cycle, oxygen is used to convert the carbon atoms of the acetyl groups into carbon dioxide and the hydrogen atoms into water. In the process, a number of small amounts of energy are released, step-by-step. These energy quanta are used to convert low-energy ADP into high-energy ATP. This ATP, analogous to a fully charged (ATP) battery, is then available to power whatever reactions are required, anywhere in this cell. It can also be exported out of the cell and used elsewhere if that is appropriate. Once it has been used and the high energy ATP battery has run down to a low energy ADP state this latter then has to return to a mitochondrion and be recharged.

Without these fully charged ATP batteries you will have very little energy.

Fats

Fatty acids are broken down in a process called beta oxidation. Unlike glucose breakdown this first step occurs not in the cytosol but, because it is an oxidation reaction, in the mitochondria or, to a lesser extent, in peroxisomes (organelles where peroxides are dealt with). This explains why, in cancer, when mitochondria are compromised, the total energy production of the cell may have to come from glucose, leading to the often quoted statement 'sugar feeds cancer'. The fatty acids are then converted into acetyl groups, which go through the Krebs cycle as before. This means that the majority of the energy derived from the fats, as well as from glucose, is released during the Krebs cycle.

From all this it is clear that the Krebs cycle is absolutely vital for your production of energy. Many different nutrients are needed as coenzymes (to help the enzymes) for this cycle to operate smoothly. They include vitamins B_2, B_3 and B_5. Trace minerals, such as magnesium, zinc and manganese are needed, both directly and indirectly. A number of toxins can interfere with the various steps around the cycle, including arsenic, antimony, mercury, fluoride and a number of toxic organic compounds. A steady supply of oxygen is essential, as is the removal of the carbon dioxide that is produced as the waste product, so make sure you breathe deeply.

The Optimum Nutrition Evaluation or ONE test (see page 95) measures the levels of different compounds that are produced and then altered within the Krebs cycle sequence. If the levels of some are too high and of others are too low then the problematic points in the cycle can be identified. Some of these problems can be due to the active interference by toxins and others may be due to a deficiency of essential nutrients. Both these faults can be corrected once they have been identified.

When the process goes wrong

The main potential danger point is the pivotal reaction from the EM pathway to a mitochondrion, and it can make the difference between a cell being healthy or becoming a cancer cell. If the acetyl group from glucose enters a mitochondrion, even if inefficiently, then you have either a healthy cell or one that is struggling and producing energy inefficiently.

If there is a blockage at this point the pyruvate molecules build up. Instead of going into the mitochondria as acetyl groups, they go sideways down the escape route and are converted into lactic acid. Lactic acid does not enter the Krebs cycle. Almost none of the body's cells can metabolise this lactate so it is exported into the boodstream and travels to the liver where, at a significant energy cost, it is rebuilt back up into glucose. This process uses up the energy that was originally obtained from the EM pathway when the glucose was initially processed. The rebuilt glucose may return to the cells and start again, along the EM pathway, but if the pivotal point is still blocked it could well keep going round in a loop, and often does just this, particularly in cancer cells.

When cells turn cancerous it is common to find there is decreased mitochondrial function, the pivotal step is blocked and there is an increased production of lactic acid. Worse still, it is l-lactic acid or left-handed lactic acid that is formed rather than the more usual d-lactic acid or the right handed form that is produced in the normal exercise fatigue of healthy cells. This l-lactic acid, produced by cells that are turning cancerous, stimulates cellular replication thereby producing more cancer cells. This failure of energy production is one of the reasons why people with cancer commonly lack energy.

If your cells are seriously deprived of oxygen over an extended period, or if any of the trace nutrients required for the function of the two pathways are missing, or if for some other reason your cells convert from the healthy aerobic breakdown of macronutrients in the mitochondria to total reliance on anaerobic fermentation in the cytosol, there will be a build up of lactic acid and cancer is a very possible consequence.

In fact it can be said that your body's way of reacting to a reduced availability of oxygen, at the tissue level, is to convert cells' healthy aerobic metabolism to unhealthy anaerobic metabolism and hence into cancer cells. This may seem absurd, but at the cellular level it can actually be seen as a survival strategy, even if the survival is only at the cellular level and a short-term solution that eventually compromises your life.

There is a further aspect to this predisposing factor here. If your Krebs cycle is not functioning correctly, at least in the cancer cells, it probably means that your mitochondria are not functioning. They may be functioning poorly, or not at all. This does more than greatly reduce your energy production. Your mitochondria play a key role in triggering apoptosis. This is the cell's decision to commit voluntary suicide, a decision usually taken by unhealthy or faulty cells. When your mitochondria are not active there is reduced apoptosis and so compromised cancer cells are free to stay alive and so to increase in number more rapidly than healthy cells with active mitochondria.

Testing for the Vital Signs

Both of the pathways of glucose breakdown can be tested.

A useful test for the level of activity of the EM pathway is to test for an enzyme in the EM pathway compound called phosphohexose isomerase or PHI. If PHI is present in higher than normal amounts it indicates excessive activity of the EM pathway, the possibility of reduced function of the mitochondria and that the cells are turning anaerobic. This test is offered by American Metabolics as part of their CA Profile.

Do the ONE test, as described on page 95, to check out your Krebs cycle and apply the treatments indicated by the results you receive.

Treatment

Follow the suggestions given in the report you receive from the ONE test. If your PHI is high you will need the help of your practitioner who will plan an appropriate treatment programme for you. It may involve doing other tests to gather more information. It will almost certainly involve eliminating sugar from your diet and increasing your intake of all the nutrients that encourage normal mitochondrial activity, including almost all the B group vitamins and several trace minerals, as already discussed.

Detecting and then correcting any faults that you may have in either the EM pathway or the Krebs cycle is an important step that contributes to your avoidance of cancer.

CHAPTER 17

Predisposing Factor No. 9 – Faulty Glucose Metabolism

In the previous chapter I described the way cells convert glucose into energy. We now need to go back a step and consider how glucose is handled from the moment you eat the initial carbohydrate until the moment the glucose molecule enters your cells.

To be healthy, and to avoid cancer, you should not eat sugars, sugar-related foods or refined carbohydrates, all of which result in sudden surges in the level of glucose in your blood. Most people know they should avoid these foods, but they find the discipline difficult. Perhaps, by the time you have read the last chapter and this one you will find the discipline is easier.

To help you understand the reasons for these dietary instructions it is important to understand how your body handles the various sugars you eat.

Normal Glucose Management

When you are healthy your normal or resting blood glucose level should remain within a concentration range of 3.0–5.5 mmol/l. When you eat foods that contain sugars or starches these release glucose, if you eat food that contains fructose or galactose (see Chapter 10) these two sugars are converted into glucose. Thus, almost all carbohydrates enter your bloodstream as glucose.

In an ideal situation, this glucose should be released slowly from your food and be only slowly absorbed into your bloodstream. Your blood glucose level would then rise, but only slightly. This rising blood glucose level should immediately trigger your pancreas to produce and mobilise the hormone insulin and release it into your bloodstream. Insulin is aided by, and dependent on, glucose tolerance factor (GTF), which contains chromium and vitamin B_3. Insulin, with the help of GTF, then triggers the cells throughout your body to take up the glucose sufficiently that your blood glucose level rapidly returns to normal.

If, at any moment, there is more glucose than your cells need, then depending on the type of cell, they either build it up into glycogen where it is stored until it is needed or they convert it into fat, which is also stored until needed.

There needs to be a counterbalance to the insulin. After all, your pancreas does not know when you will stop eating carbohydrates and the influx of glucose will stop, and so it inevitably overshoots the mark, and your blood glucose level starts to fall below the normal range. Other hormones then come into play, including glucagon, also from your pancreas, and adrenalin, from your adrenal glands. These stimulate a rise in the level of glucose in your blood, until it is brought back up to normal. Between these various hormones, the normal balance is restored.

You may have heard of foods having a high or low glycemic index. This is a measure of the height to which they raise your blood glucose level. If you eat a diet of foods with a high-glycemic index – refined carbohydrates such as white flour, white pasta and white rice, or potatoes, parsnips and bananas, or sugar itself in any of its many forms – glucose will enter your bloodstream faster than your insulin can deal with it or that your healthy cells can accept it. For a period of time, before the insulin gets things back under control, your blood glucose level will be significantly above the normal level. This is a danger time. It can cause or be indicative of a number of health problems, including diabetes. A prolonged high blood glucose level is a predisposing factor to cancer.

If you have any cancer cells present, this period of high blood glucose level will constitute a bonanza period for them and encourage them into further activity and replication, as I will explain later in this chapter. This is one of the reasons why faulty glucose metabolism is a predisposing factor.

Hypoglycaemia, or Low Blood Glucose Level

Many people eating a diet full of high-glycemic foods are also under stress and at risk of adrenal exhaustion (see Chapter 20). When this happens the blood glucose level goes up after eating, insulin pushes it down, but there is a delayed response from your exhausted adrenal glands so your blood glucose level remains low. The result is extended periods of low blood glucose levels (hypoglycaemia) before things can return to normal.

This state generates a range of physical and emotional symptoms including fatigue, the jitters, irritability, sugar cravings, the shakes and more. Partly, these symptoms are due to the fact that your brain, in the short term, is totally dependent on glucose for energy. Unlike the cells elsewhere in your body, your brain cells do not use fats for energy unless they are glucose-starved for three days or more. This means that the minute your blood glucose level falls below normal your brain is not being fed, it behaves badly, and the symptoms already mentioned are the result. Unfortunately, most people's response to these symptoms is to eat more sugar, or sugary foods, and so aggravate the problem.

Hypoglycaemia is often an undiagnosed problem and it is not until it leads to diabetes that its existence is recognised. Since it can lead to diabetes, hypoglycaemia too can be considered to be a predisposing factor.

Hyperglycaemia, or Diabetes

At least two problems combine to convert **hypo**glycaemia into diabetes (or **hyper**glycaemia).

On the one hand, these huge demands on pancreatic insulin output begin to cause pancreatic exhaustion and insulin insufficiency. This will be made worse if you are zinc deficient, as this mineral is needed for the production of the active form of insulin.

On the other hand, your cells gradually become resistant to insulin and so more insulin than normal is needed to drive the glucose into your cells. This can be triggered or aggravated if you are deficient in chromium (and hence GTF),[78] vanadium[79] and many of the other B-group vitamins. (In fact many other deficiencies can contribute to both of these problems, but that discussion would take us away from our main focus.) This is yet another reason why nutrient deficiencies (see Chapters 11 and 12) are considered to be predisposing factors; predisposing, this time, to diabetes, which in turn is a predisposing factor to cancer.[80]

There are several reasons for this, but the most obvious one is that people with diabetes, by definition, have prolonged periods of high blood glucose levels and this glucose feeds cancer cells.[81] It is thought that we all produce cancer cells frequently, possibly every day, but our immune system generally deals with them. Having excess glucose in your bloodstream only makes this job more difficult. (There are other reasons why this is a problem, but these get us into more technical areas and are covered in the second book in this series, *Cancer Concerns.*)

The net result of this, in terms of a named disease, is that you become diabetic. This is generally managed by (a) dietary modifications; (b) drugs to stabilise your blood glucose level; or (c) insulin. Some people with diabetes have a normal output of insulin but their cells are non-responsive, hence the use of additional insulin as a treatment. It's a sort of sledgehammer approach. It is a pity that diabetics are not given the necessary nutrients that would make things easier for their own insulin to work.

The consequences of diabetes

Many people to whom I have spoken feel, or have been told by their doctors, that as long as their blood glucose level does not rise too far above normal, there is little to worry about; however, the long-term consequences of diabetes are kidney damage and increased urinary frequency, deteriorating eyesight, worsening circulation with possible gangrene, heart problems and cancer – not such small problems.

To claim that diabetes has reached epidemic proportions is not too much of an exaggeration. Its incidence is rising so rapidly that if it were an infectious disease the current situation would certainly be called an epidemic. This is particularly true in Western countries such as the UK and the USA; it is also true on a world scale. It is estimated that worldwide 124 million people were diabetic in 1997 and that by 2010 the incidence will have nearly doubled to closer to 221 million.[82]

How did diabetes become so common, and what are the consequences? There are many causes, but a lot of the problems can be placed at the door of the general rise in the combined consumption of both sugar and refined carbohydrates, associated with the fall in the amount of B vitamins, chromium and vanadium in the diet. The latter is due to increased consumption of processed foods and to poor food choices in general. These nutrients tend to be in whole-grain products and vegetables and few people eat sufficient of these foods. In addition, the minerals can only be present in the food if the food is grown on mineral-rich soil, and these two minerals are rarely added back to the soil in commercial farming. Added to this there are the high stress levels that most people put themselves under, the adrenal exhaustion that can result, and the strain that is put on the pancreas by today's bad diet of foods such as overheated fats, trans-fatty acids and an excessive intake of proteins in relation to fruits and vegetables.

Even soy puts a strain on the pancreas as, like other dried beans and their products, it contains an anti-nutritive factor. This factor inhibits trypsin, one of the pancreatic enzymes used for protein digestion, thus making the pancreas work harder to produce a sufficient amount of enzymes to digest the high protein meal. Keep in mind, also, that many meat products are now 'extended' with additions of textured vegetable protein derived largely from soy. Read the labels. You may be surprised to find how many foods contain soy. To balance these statements, there is evidence that fermented soy products such as tempeh and miso, do not contain this factor and may be beneficial foods.[83]

Glucose and Cancer Cells

Cancer cells are sugar hungry. Sugar feeds cancer. Technically, 'cancer is an obligate sugar metaboliser'.[84] According to double Nobel laureate Dr Linus Pauling in a personal communication, 'Sugar is the most hazardous foodstuff in the American diet.'

A correlation has been reported between high sugar intake and mortality from breast cancer in post-menopausal women.[85] The authors go on to state that 'A possible connecting link between sugar consumption and breast cancer is insulin. This is an absolute requirement for the proliferation of normal mammary tissue and experimental mammary tumours may regress in its absence.'

Cancer cells use sugar very wastefully. Frequently, they are found to be operating on the EM pathway only and not the Krebs cycles, thus they need huge amounts of glucose. To ensure an adequate supply, and that they have a competitive edge for it over healthy cells, cancer cells have a huge number of receptor sites, or entrances, for glucose; for example, 'Cancer cells demonstrate a 3 to 5 fold increase in glucose uptake compared to healthy cells.'[86] Other estimates put this at between six and 30 times as many receptor sites as are found on healthy cells; for example, '23 times as many'[87] or 'Cancer cells have six times as many receptor sites for insulin (and hence glucose uptake) as healthy cells'.[88] Whatever the correct figure, cancer cells have a huge competitive advantage in the rush for glucose. There has even been research into ways to block this glucose availability or uptake as a form of treatment for cancer.[89] The problem with that, however, is that healthy cells also need glucose but remain less successful at getting it than are the cancer cells.

Since there is evidence that a diet that increases your blood glucose level increases your risk of developing cancer,[90] it is clear that sugar and glucose are part of this serious predisposing factor.

Not only do cancer cells have more receptor (uptake) sites than do healthy cells for glucose but they also have devised another clever tool to take in glucose and feed their insatiable appetite for it. They have developed special channels called epidermal growth factor receptors (EGFR) that stabilise a protein that channels a constant supply of glucose into the cancer cells.[91]

Furthermore, not only are cancer cells hungry for sugar, but you will also recall that the abundant supply of sugar leads cancer cells to produce harmful waste products, such as l-lactic acid, which further encourages the growth of more cancer cells (explained in Chapter 16).

All this should warn you, loud and clear, that sugar feeds cancer; you should avoid eating sugar in all its forms; you should avoid food with a high glycemic index, including refined white flour and white rice; you should correct any problems you may have with your management of sugar metabolism.

I put this somewhat more graphically to one patient who had not got the point in previous consultations and was still eating ice cream and bars of chocolate. 'Imagine', I said, 'that your cells are like beggars, begging for food. Cancer cells have a huge begging bowl; healthy cells have small ones. If a small amount of food (glucose in our scenario) is delivered at spaced intervals, all the cells can get a small amount and can do so at a steady rate. If a large amount is delivered all at one time the beggars with small bowls can only take up a small amount, but the beggars with large bowls can gorge on the excess. They become the successful cells, and so cancer develops further.

Every time you eat sugar you are feeding the cancer,' I said, in order to drive the point home. It is no wonder that you feel exhausted, but the cancer thrives. You need to provide energy for your healthy cells from different sources, from fats and slow-release carbohydrates such as vegetables, not from a large and sudden influx of glucose from sugar-laden chocolates and ice cream.

On today's diet, with a high content of high glycemic foods and a generally inadequate supply of micronutrients, including trace minerals, it is common to find that more and more people, as they age, are developing both hypoglycaemia and maturity-onset diabetes.[92] In this way they also increase their risk of developing cancer.

More on glucose and cancer

Space precludes a more detailed discussion, but here are some points to consider:

- Free glucose in the bloodstream attaches to (glycosylates) proteins, thus impeding their reactions.
- Sugar encourages the growth of yeasts and moulds, including but not limited to *Candida albicans.*
- Sugar reduces immune function, which leads to increased infections and increased risk of cancer.[93]
- Increased sugar intake increases insulin output, and insulin is a risk factor for cancer.[94]
- The sugar-induced increased insulin output increases the production of the pro-inflammatory and pro-thrombotic prostaglin PG2 series. (Note: omega-3 oils, from fish, evening primrose and borage oils, lead to the anti-inflammatory, anti-thrombotic prostaglandin PG3 series.)

Sugar and vitamin C

The chemical formulae for glucose and vitamin C are so similar that cancer cells absorb the latter in far larger quantities than do healthy cells, to the detriment of the cancer cells; however, if your blood glucose level is high, this competes with the vitamin C and the absorption of the latter, by the cancer cells, is reduced.

PET scans make use of the uptake of glucose by cancer cells. Fluorodeoxyglucose, or FDG, is an analogue of glucose. It is taken up preferentially by cells that use increased amounts of glucose and is frequently used as the tracer prior to a PET scan for cancer. It accumulates in cancerous tissue but is then unable to leave the cells. The radioactive fluoride isotope within the molecule can then be detected during the scan and the tumour located.

On the bright side, mannoheptulose, a seven-carbon sugar found in avocado pears, reduces the uptake of glucose by cancer cells, so enjoy this delicious, low-carbohydrate food.[95]

Testing for the Vital Signs

This process, the progression from health through hypoglycaemia to diabetes, can be both detected and stopped at any point along the progression. The sooner you do this the better.

Glucose tolerance test

The glucose tolerance test involves having your blood glucose level measured at the start of the test, then drinking a sugar-rich solution and monitoring your blood glucose level. Ideally this monitoring should be done every 30 minutes for the next six hours, although doctors usually do it once an hour for three hours, as they are generally looking only for the possibility of diabetes, not for hypoglycaemia. This complete test will show you just how well or how poorly your body is managing your blood glucose level and how rapidly your blood glucose level returns to normal after the sugar challenge. If the level of insulin in your blood is measured each time you measure the amount of glucose, you will get even more useful information.

If this test shows a short period of increased blood glucose level followed by an extended period of low blood glucose level, often accompanied by unpleasant symptoms, you should recognise this as hypoglycaemia and start to treat and correct that before anything worse develops. If the results show an unusually high spike in your blood glucose level, before it falls back to, and perhaps below, normal, you could be in a transition phase between hypoglycaemia and diabetes. If your blood glucose level rises and stays high from the start, falling back towards the normal level only slowly, you could already be diabetic. All these situations should be corrected. They are all serious predisposing factors and if ignored may lead you to far more serious problems.

In practical terms it is possible for you to do this test at home, using the equipment that diabetics use to monitor their blood glucose level; however, I strongly advise against this. There is the possibility that at some time during the test your blood glucose level could fall so low that you faint. The level at which this could occur varies, but below 3.0 mmol/l is already too low for some people. Such a drop is a situation that diabetics recognise as 'having a hypo'. If a professional is monitoring your test procedure they will almost certainly abort the test if your level falls too low or if your symptoms suggest that you should do this. The solution, if such a hypo does occur, is of course, to have some fruit or something that will raise your blood glucose level safely back up to normal. This will abort the test early but it will, by definition, mean that you have already shown yourself to be hypoglycaemic, with or without a prior period of hyperglycaemia,

If you already know you have cancer, or if cancer is strongly suspected, it would not be wise for you to do this test, as the high sugar intake would feed any cancer cells present. If you have cancer, you should certainly assume that sugar is a problem and sugar management is important. You should eat only low-glycemic foods.

HbA1C

To avoid the glucose tolerance test but to test for diabetes, there is another test you can do. This is based on the fact that some of the glucose molecules in your blood attach themselves to your haemoglobin (found inside your red blood cells), forming a compound called HbA1C.

The half-life of your red blood cells is 60 days. This means that after 60 days half of your red blood cells, with their associated HbA1C, have died and an equal number of new ones, with no HbA1C, have been produced and sent out from your bone marrow. As a result, there is a normal, steady concentration of HbA1C that is expected to be present in your blood. For every moment that your blood glucose level is above normal, additional glucose molecules attach themselves to your haemoglobin, and they remain attached, even when your blood glucose level returns to normal. As a result, your level of HbA1C will rise above normal. This means that by having a blood sample tested for the amount of HbA1C it contains you can find out whether or not your blood has, at varying times, carried an excess of glucose and if you are becoming, or are, diabetic.

Your Optimising Strategy

At the risk of sounding repetitive, the treatment involves avoiding all the foods with a high-glycemic index and making sure that you have an adequate intake of the vitamins and minerals already mentioned that are required for glucose metabolism. A very useful website for further information on this is www.glycemicindex.com, an online GI database developed and regularly updated by the University of Sydney.

In addition, and certainly if you have, or suspect, cancer, you should not drink fruit juices, as they are a concentrated source of fruit sugar and you should probably not eat fruit on its own, other than berries. Berries are exempt from this general embargo because they are relatively low in sugar, and they contain high levels of ellagic acid, resveratrol, salvesterols and many other beneficial phytonutrients that are protective against cancer, so the pay off is worth it. Root vegetable juices, such as carrot or beetroot, contain beneficial carotenes and other compounds, but they are also high in sugar and so these should be combined with much larger amounts of vegetable juice derived from above-ground vegetables.

All of this is good advice, whether or not you have cancer and whether or not you choose to follow the MDS treatments for cancer as well as the CAM therapies.

———

If you do nothing else, if you decide there is only one lifestyle change you will make to avoid cancer and improve your health, make it this: give up sugar, in all its forms, in anything.

CHAPTER 18

Predisposing Factor No. 10 – Faulty Neurotransmitters

We have discussed diet, nutrition and digestion, your liver and toxins, energy production and the management of glucose. It is time now to consider your body as a whole, and we will start with a discussion of the way your brain communicates with your cells and how communications occur through the immensely complex entity that is your body. If there are faults in the way this overall system is managed, they constitute a strong predisposing factor for a range of health problems and can certainly lead into the full cancer process.

What Neurotransmitters Do

To understand how the communications work, it is necessary to consider the actions at the cellular level. Many of the cells in your body are separated from each other by a small gap, called the synaptic gap. These gaps exist between one nerve cell and the next, and between a nerve cell and an adjacent muscle cell. For communication from your brain to reach any other part of your body, the message has to travel a significant distance. The message is first passed by the release of a small molecule called a neurotransmitter (literally something that transmits from one neuron, or nerve cell, to the next) from the last nerve cell within your brain to the first nerve cell outside your brain. From there a chemical change ripples along the membrane or wall of this first nerve cell to the end of the cell's arm, known as the axon. Here it triggers the release of another neurotransmitter. There are many different neurotransmitters. They include compounds such as acetylcholine, GABA, dopamine, adrenalin, noradrenalin and serotonin.

Once a neurotransmitter has been released, it travels across the tiny synaptic gap and is picked up by a receptor site on the target cell. This receptor site is usually a protein either on the surface of, or embedded through, the membrane of the target cell. Once this neurotransmitter is received, it crosses the membrane, enters the target cell and triggers the next electrical ripple along the length of the second nerve cell. For this nerve cell to communicate with the target muscle, another chemical neurotransmitter, possibly a different one, is then released and jumps across the synaptic gap to the muscle cell, which then responds with the appropriate movement. For the target muscle cell to acknowledge or receive the neurotransmitter it too has to have the appropriate receptor site already built in.

Here is an example, to make it clearer. Your brain feels an emotion such as fear. It needs to move your body. The emotion and the thought stimulate your brain cells, via neurotransmitters, to pass this message to a nerve that runs down to your leg muscles and instructs your leg to move, perhaps to run or fight. The emotion triggered the action via the neurotransmitters. We can generalise on this. Thoughts trigger the emotions that send out messages that then stimulate actions. In this way your brain communicates with the rest of your body via chemicals called neurotransmitters.

So far we have talked of your brain communicating with your muscles, but there is more, as we shall see.

How your thoughts and feelings affect your health

It was first thought that these molecules, manufactured within brain cells, were the messengers only to the next nerve cell or to the cells of the individual muscle that a particular nerve activated. In other words, it was thought that only neurons and muscle cells had receptor sites able to receive the neurotransmitter message.

Now, after the work of Candace Pert, described in her book *Molecules of Emotion*,[96] and other researchers like her, we know that there are receptor sites for neurotransmitters on the cells of your immune system. (Candace Pert was formerly Research Professorship in the Department of Physiology and Biophysics at Georgetown University School of Medicine in Washington, DC, and is currently the Scientific Director of RAPID Pharmaceuticals, Inc.) This is an amazing discovery with huge implications. Put simply, this means that your thoughts and the activity of your brain and the cells within it can send messages, or 'talk' directly to your immune system via chemical pathways and thus affect the way you handle the risk or the occurrence of infections. It is almost a commonplace that when a much-loved partner of several decades dies, the remaining and deeply saddened partner soon develops an infection, such as pneumonia, and often also dies. They are said to have pined away. We now know, at the chemical level, how this can have happened. The emotions have affected, adversely in this case, the way the person's brain communicates with the immune system, and the immune system, as a result, has failed to function with its usual efficiency.

There is more. We now know that your hormonal glands (the glands that produce and send out the hormones that dictate so many of your body's reactions) also have receptor sites for these neurotransmitters. This is another exciting discovery. It means that your brain and your thoughts can influence the way your endocrine system (where hormones are produced) performs and affect the target tissues of these hormones.

Your thoughts affect your whole body

Finally, and as a logical extension of these discoveries, it is thought probable that all the tissues in your body, certainly your major organs, have such receptor sites, and so their functions too are affected by your thoughts and your brain activity. Keep this in mind as you read through the rest of this book and particularly Chapters 19 and 20 which explain the way in which your thoughts and emotions can affect your whole body.

Many people have argued against these connections for decades, or longer, but it is becoming increasingly difficult, if not impossible, to maintain that thoughts do not affect the way your body functions, whether good or bad, and therefore your health. At the experiential level you know this. You know, for instance, that if you imagine doing something or you think about a situation that frightens you, you can feel your adrenalin pumping, your heart rate increasing and your hands sweating, even when you are sitting in safety. Think of lemon juice and your saliva will run. These are all physiological responses to a thought.

This knowledge of neurotransmitters and the existence of receptor sites found all over your body has huge implications. It is the physiological and biochemical underpinning for our growing understanding that your thoughts and feelings can act directly on your body. They do this by the type and quantity of the neurotransmitters that are sent out from the brain, and these neurotransmitters carry their messages throughout your body. The neurotransmitters are either stimulatory or inhibitory, they either turn an action on or they turn it off, and as such they dictate the response of the target cells and tissues.

The recognition of this physiological link between thoughts and emotions on the one hand and your body's physiological changes on the other adds weight to the idea that your thoughts have a direct effect on your health, and that thinking and psychotherapy are important and have an enormous amount to offer as powerful healing procedures. This is the topic for the next chapter.

At the purely physiological level, you need to have the correct output and ratio of all the neurotransmitters to ensure optimum function of your immune system, your hormone or endocrine system and the various other organs and systems throughout your body. By determining your level of the various neurotransmitters you can learn where there are imbalances, deficiencies and excesses. By correcting these you can improve your overall health in very many different ways. By doing this you will be removing some of the predisposing factors and so, according to the thesis proposed in this book, stepping backwards along the cancer process.

Testing for the Vital Signs

The levels of your neurotransmitters can be tested by a urine sample that you can post to the testing laboratory. Several groups of compounds can be tested for:

- The levels of the neurotransmitters themselves.
- The levels of precursors – the substances from which the neurotransmitters are made. Examples of these include tryptophan, or 5-HTP, which is needed for the production of serotonin, and the amino acids tyrosine and phenylalanine, which are needed for the production of adrenalin, noradrenalin, thyroxine and dopamine. Clearly, if such precursor deficiencies

are recognised, this provides clues as to why the neurotransmitter itself is in short supply and indicates the most appropriate therapy.

- The levels of the compounds produced by the neurotransmitters after their activity has taken place, which will provide more useful information. The details of this are complex and should be discussed with your practitioner.

- The levels of a variety of neurotoxins – substances that are toxic to the nervous system. One such toxin is indican, which has already been discussed in relation to colon toxins in Chapter 13. Other toxins can cause increased free-radical activity (toxicity) in the brain, or they can show the possible presence of moulds or fungi, or of bacterial or other infections.

George S

George was in good general health but had trouble maintaining body weight and was concerned about the toxins in his environment. He had seen an apparently healthy friend suddenly develop cancer and was keen to make sure that he was not heading in the same direction.

He did the neurotransmitter test as part of a general check-up. The tests relating specifically to Phase Two of the cancer process showed normal results, which was a relief and a reassurance to him; however, his neurological profile showed the presence of high levels of phthalates. These are environmental toxins that can enter the brain and act as neurotoxins, working against other needed neurotransmitters. They are used as plasticisers and are found in and on many of the plastic containers used for food and drink. So I advised George to stop consuming foods from plastic containers, especially fatty foods such as butter-like spreads, vegetable oils, or take-away meals, and not to drink liquids, including mineral water, from plastic bottles. As always, it is impossible, in individual cases, to know what you have prevented, but eliminating toxins from your lifestyle and body is an important aspect of preventing health problems.

Your Optimising Strategy

Clearly this whole topic is complex. It is certainly one for which you will want professional guidance, but it is also one you should know about and follow up on. Some laboratories that provide the tests will tell you which amino acids and the dosages they think you should take to correct your neurotransmitter balance. They can also supply the products they think you need (see Resources: Neuroscience). Although you could do this on your own, you are likely to do a lot better if you enlist the help of a practitioner who not only has access to these results but also to the results of other tests you may have had done, and will compile details of your diet and lifestyle and a knowledge of whatever symptoms you have. Other laboratories will give general guidance and suggest a wider range of remedies (see Resources: Neuro Lab Limited), but you will almost certainly need advice as to how to implement such a regime.

Most, although not all, neurotransmitters are made of, or from, amino acids. This means that a deficiency of an individual neurotransmitter will often tell you which amino acids are needed to correct a problem. In addition, you will need the co-factors that are required to catalyse the production or function of that neurotransmitter as it may be a lack of these that has caused the imbalance. Vitamin B_6 is essential to the metabolism of all amino acids, but several other nutrients are required as well, depending on the neurotransmitter in question.

If compounds are found that increase or reflect increased free-radical activity in your brain, you will need to increase your intake of antioxidants in general and those that cross the blood–brain barrier (BBB) in particular. Melatonin is particularly good, but unfortunately is not available in the UK, although it is in the US and on the Internet. You can increase your own production of melatonin by sleeping in a totally dark room. That means ensuring that there is no light seeping round or though the curtains, no red 'stand-by' lights on any items of electrical equipment and, if you have to get up to go to the toilet during the night, doing so in the dark. If you absolutely have to put the light on to do this, use a torch with a red bulb, this red light slows melatonin production down less than the light from normal light bulbs. If your melatonin-producing switch has been turned off by bright light, it will take a while to turn it back on and you may well be getting up by then, so your

production of melatonin can be seriously disrupted by sleep disturbances that expose you to light.

Other beneficial antioxidants that cross the BBB include the proanthocyanidins and anthocyanins, some of the subgroups of compounds
collectively referred to as bioflavonoids. They are generally found in
deeply coloured fruits, usually red ones, including red grapes, and in
many brightly coloured vegetables. Other beneficial compounds that
cross the BBB are MSM, commonly used in supplements aimed at reducing the pain of arthritis, and R-lipoic acid (which is better than the more
commonly available alpha-lipoic acid), also the herb artemesia, especially in the form of artemesinin, which is known to be beneficial in the
treatment of cancer.[97]

NeuroScience Inc. (www.neurorelief.com) in the USA offers a simple
neurotransmitter profile based on urine analysis. It provides a report
and a suggested list of remedial supplements, which it also provides.
Neuro Lab Limited in the UK provides a more in-depth neurotransmitter
profile, but your practitioner will need to help you to make full use of the
results of its test.

In this chapter we covered the known and incontrovertible link between
the internal activity of your brain or thoughts and emotions, on the one
side, and the physical manifestations of these throughout your body, on
the other, via known messenger molecules. It is now time to follow this up
further.

CHAPTER 19

Predisposing Factor No. 11 – Stress and Emotional Issues

So far we have talked about physical and chemical problems that are predisposing factors for cancer. Now it is time to talk about stress and the impact it can have on your body and the way it can predispose you to cancer. In Chapter 20 we will then focus on your adrenal glands, the organs that have a major role to play in the way your body handles stress.

The Outcome of Stress

It is common to find that people who develop cancer have experienced unusual or heavy stress a few years prior to their diagnosis, about two years on average, although there is considerable variation.[98] Stress puts an immense pressure on your adrenal glands and on many other parts of your body. Your thoughts and emotions have immense power over the state of your body and so on your health. The good news is that, just as thoughts and emotions can cause ill health, so too can they assist in your recovery when appropriately handled.[99]

It is unfortunate that we have to use the word 'stress'. Even Hans Selye who, back in the middle of the last century, was the first to recognise and describe the stress response, soon came to regret his use of the word, because it has two meanings:

1   Stress is applied pressure, or push to change. In this sense going on holiday is a stress, as is any action you take other than, arguably, lying supine. Every move you make or any emotion you feel, or any thought you think, applies some stressor to your body. There is no value judgement implied by this use of the

term, it is merely a recognition of the forces applied, regardless of whether they are pleasant or unpleasant, good or bad. We will refer to this as 'good or neutral stress'. This is an important aspect to grasp, as you will see.

or

2 Stress is something bad that causes you pain, discomfort or problems. In this use of the term there is an implied pejorative connotation to the term. This is the most common use of the term, but for our purposes here we will call this 'bad stress'.

Bad Stress

We have seen from the previous chapter the deeply significant mechanisms that can forge links between your mind and emotions on the one hand and your body on the other, and hence the potential impact of your emotions and mental state on your health and the possible development of cancer. Bad stress increases your requirement for certain nutrients, reduces the oxygen supply to your tissues, can trigger the change from aerobic to anaerobic metabolism (explained in Chapter 16) and increases the possible production of harmful l-lactic acid (also in Chapter 16).

Bad stressful states can alter the flow of your digestive juices and the production of digestive enzymes, thus interfering with digestion and leading to the possible development of pathogens in your digestive tract. Worries and concerns can change your brain chemistry, which in turn can change the messages that are sent to the cells of your immune system and hormone glands. We know that when you smile your white blood cells become more active and go to work attacking foreign invaders. When you are sad and frown, however, their activity decreases – so smile! It not only makes you feel good, regardless of what is going on in your life at the moment, but it also helps you to stay healthy.

Heavy-duty bad stress (emotional) and overload (stress caused by physical exhaustion and burnout) frequently lead to a lack of care, lack of time for a good diet, failure to take supplements or exercise, or to make time for rest and emotional warmth and joy. This further increases your risk of developing a variety of health problems, including cancer.

The worst type of stress is the helpless and hopeless variety, when you feel trapped in a situation for which you can see no positive outcome; for example, the mother of toddler-aged children may be desperate to get out of her marriage but feels she could not possibly cope with the children on her own; a man may be working for a boss he dislikes, who is manipulative or unethical, but he cannot leave because his family depends on his income or on the reference he would need (but would not get) if he resigned. These situations can eat away at you, making you feel helpless and hopeless, and stuck in a situation you feel you cannot change.

Wendy S

Wendy was a successful career woman in her fifties. Childless, she lived near her parents, for whom she cared and with whom she was close. When they were killed in a car crash she was bereft. She had lost her emotional anchor and compensated for this by throwing herself into activities relating to the property and assets she had inherited. Unwisely, she accepted a business proposition from a man with no assets but, he claimed, many skills appropriate for the proposed project. She would be the silent partner providing the needed resources; he would perform. He did not perform. As the months went by she became incensed by the deceits, half-truths and pretences that were used to cover up his many incompetences, and overloaded by the onerous additional demands made on her time as she tried to keep the whole project going, as well as her career. It was, she told me, like trying to run through knee-high muddy clay. A truthful and accurate woman, Wendy lost touch with any certainty as she kept hearing the ever more extraordinary, and seemingly plausible, tales he was telling her colleagues. This is bad stress, stress of the type in which the individual is both overloaded and feels helpless as to making a positive change and hopeless as to the outcome or ending of the situation.

In the end, Wendy engineered the departure of her business partner, then coped as best she could and retrieved what was possible of the business; however, the damage had been done. Two years later she was diagnosed with a fast-growing cancer and was told she would be dead within the next 18 months to two years, even with radical medical treatment – treatment that she refused. She preferred to place her trust in the CAM therapies instead. When we tested her adrenal glands – the ones that help you handle stress, good or bad – they were running on negative; when we did the ONE test (explained on page 95) for her she was deficient in almost all nutrients, in spite of the good diet she had been on and all the supplements she had been taking. She set to doing all the tests described here and righting the wrongs that showed up.

However, it is much easier to prevent a problem than to treat it. Wendy would have been wise to get out of the situation sooner. Unfortunately, once you have developed cancer, removing the stressor is not enough, as cancer, once established, is self-perpetuating, so you still have the mountain to climb of beating the cancer. Even dealing with the residual emotions is not enough, although this is a vital part of recovery. A full treatment programme is necessary and this, at the time of writing, several years from the start, she is still working on.

It is all too easy, if you are of that temperament, to think that you are invincible, that you have coped so far, and that you can continue to cope. You can't. Eventually the tank will be empty. As humans, we evolved to produce large spurts of energy and activity as we dealt with the beasts of the forest, then periods of quiet and recovery when we returned to our caves. It is stupid, not heroic, to keep performing miracles, just because you can.

Cancer and our emotional needs

Bad stress can take other forms; they may be much less dramatic, yet they too can be predisposing factors for cancer. People who endure long-term chronic bad stress can become ill. They may hide their feelings; the stressor may seem slight to other people but be of major significance to the individual.

Like many CAM psychotherapists, I have worked with clients who have become ill, even to the extent of developing cancer, which was helped immensely when their emotional needs were met; almost as if it was their body's way of crying for help.

Davina R

Davina was a grandmother when she came to see me. The eldest of five children she had grown up hearing herself praised for all she did for her siblings. As an adult she became the focus of the rest of the family, she looked after the nephews and nieces, and then the grandchildren. She was always there. As we worked together, she suddenly came to realise that she felt, subconsciously, that she was not loved for herself, but for what she did for others, and so she had to keep doing it. By the age of 68 and widowed she was exhausted. She needed to receive as well as to give, yet she 'knew' that if she stopped giving she would be unloved and alone. She developed arthritis and other health problems, but still coped, and was still praised for what she was doing for others, in spite of her own problems. Then she developed cancer. Finally, the family had to stop and think about her. At the unconscious level, cancer had been an (emotionally) safe way of getting her needs meet, even if it was at the possible cost of her (physical) life. After a few psychotherapy sessions she came to understand all this consciously. Although it required a lot of courage, she made a number of changes, putting her needs first, being willing to ask for and receive help, and gradually developing a balance in her emotional life.

There may be some debate about the fundamental issue in Davina's story. Yes, arguably, she had allowed herself to develop cancer. Perhaps she had eaten badly, or included many of the other predisposing factors in her lifestyle. She may even have done this, feeling it was more important to put other people's needs before her own, as part of her general strategy to gain love and approval. She was afraid of losing their approval, but by having cancer and a cast-iron need for them to look after her rather than the other way around, she had found a safe way of getting her emotional needs met.

However, there is another important issue to consider here. Being at cause does not mean being at fault. What she did was not wrong. Whole books have been written on the link between the emotions and physical health. My own book, *Choosing Health Intentionally* covers this topic from the emotional level. As we have seen with Davina, deteriorating health can be used as a way of getting your emotional needs meet.[100] This is not stupid. It is done totally unconsciously, and it is appropriate in a society where we give much more care and concern to people who are physically ill than to those who are discontented or unhappy with their life. Think of the times you may have wished you had an excuse sufficient to claim a sick-day so that you could relax, unwind, do something pleasant or take time out for yourself, and you will know what I mean.

Following psychotherapy sessions, many patients have in fact come to recognise these connections. Sometimes they can then act positively on what they have learned and use the information to make positive changes in their life. At other times, even knowing what underlies their problem does not mean they are willing to make the changes necessary for recovery. Adele is a case in point:

Adele P

When Adele came to me, she had been diagnosed with breast cancer. She had had surgery but was refusing any further treatment. She wanted a psychotherapy session. It turned out that her husband had been having an affair. When she found out about it she was furious and told him so. He said he was sorry for distressing her and agreed to end the affair, which in fact, for geographical reasons, was coming to an end anyway. Two years later she developed a lump in her breast. During the psychotherapy session she came to realise that by having breast cancer she was able to show him what distress he had caused her. I suggested that now she recognised the cause, she might feel free to move ahead and have treatment, be it MDS or CAM treatment, and might then get better. Her immediate response of, 'But if I get better he will have got away with it' showed her need to go on having it as a rod to beat him with. I did not see her again and so do not know what action she took.

How to defuse bad stress

Dealing with, and defusing, bad stress may be a lot easier than you think. In *From Stress to Success* I have described dozens of ways of dealing with bad stress. This covers both stressful situations and stressful states of mind, for the two are often not the same.

If you are in a situation that you find enormously stressful, there are several things you can do. The first avenue to explore involves ways to get out of it, either by changing the nature of the situation or by leaving it. The other avenue is to consider how you can change your attitude to it.

There is no such thing as 'a stress', separate from the individual. There are situations that you personally find stressful. Speaking in public is not, in itself, stressful. You stand up, you speak. What is stressful is what you are telling yourself other people may be thinking about how you look or perform. This makes little sense, since you will never actually know what they think, even in spite of whatever they actually say to you. The flip side of this is that some people actually love speaking in public. So it cannot be the activity itself that is stressful; therefore, it must be your thoughts in relation to it. Flying in an aeroplane is not stressful. You get in, sit back and relax, land and get out again. But if your thoughts take you on visits to all of the air crashes you have heard of, that is stressful. It is your thoughts that do it, not the event. Read my book on the subject, above all, do the exercises in my book, for it is only by doing the mental exercises that you can really make progress. Do the same with all the other books out there on similar aspects of the problem.

Learn to relax

This may be easier said than done when or if you have just been diagnosed with cancer, or if you are actively afraid you may be developing cancer. However, it is important. Some people try to meditate, others say they can't keep their mind still. You were given a good mind, so making it go blank may not be all it is cracked up to be; however, it is unhelpful to have it spinning round in uncontrolled circles. There are some simple techniques, such as EFT – the Emotional Freedom Technique[101] – and Autogenic Training[102] that can be done in just a few minutes each day and yet achieve excellent results. Most of my patients find that either or both are helpful. They are both worth exploring and you can do them on your own, at home, in your own time.

Make changes. Many people with cancer, or who have had cancer, have been able to turn it into a positive experience. They report that they have found it to be, or have been able to make it into, an amazingly constructive time, a time of learning and developing in spite of the underlying fears and problems – one that has led to many positive lifestyle changes. It is as if having cancer has given them the freedom to change their lives and to do things they would not otherwise have thought of doing. After all, if they only have a limited time left, they want to make the most of it. None of us can know when our lives might change through death, accident or financial disaster. Yet we mostly assume things will continue. You decide not go on the cruise that you would love, because paying off the mortgage or saving for your retirement seems more important, yet where is the joy you could experience and share? You don't follow your chosen ambition because the family might not approve, but who gives them the right to dictate to you? You stick to a boring job because you need to pay the school fees, yet perhaps the children would be happier and do better at school if they had a better relationship with a happier parent. Now, suddenly, once you have been diagnosed with cancer, the future could be limited. Saving for a possibly non-existent future, trying to please people when you may not be around them much longer or missing out on the good times with your children makes no sense. Maybe this is an indication that you should make some serious changes in your life.

Your Own MOT

I often suggest that patients do some or all of the following exercises:

1 List everything you would like to do in your life, but aren't doing at all or are not doing for enough of the time.

2 List everything in your life that makes your heart sing. Then ask yourself: what percentage of your life is filled by these things?

3 List all the things you do that are tedious, boring, deadening or uninteresting. What percentage of your life is filled by these things?

4 You have ten minutes to describe the life you would consider to be perfect. No restrictions. You can include things you already

have or are doing as well as things you would like to have or to
be doing.

5   Imagine you could start your life over again. Go back to the start
of your life. What things would you do differently?

Now go back to the first two lists and for each item you would like to
be doing, ask yourself:

- What have I done to be able to do this?
- What else could I do to make this possible?
- What would happen if I did make these changes?
- What stops me?
- What will happen if I don't make these changes?
- What am I now willing to do to change?
- What do these answers say about me?

Now work on the third list, the boring list, and ask yourself:

- Why do I keep doing what I don't enjoy?
- Are these activities really essential?
- If they are, how could I make them more enjoyable?
- How could I change my attitude to them?
- If they are not essential, what can I do to change them?
- What have I done to make any of these changes?
- What could I do to make any of these changes?
- What do these answers say about me?

Now, number four. Beside each item, on a scale of one to ten,
mark how much of each goal or desire you already have in your life.
Look at the figure as a percentage of the total. Is that enough? You may
be in for some surprises. You may find that you actually do have almost
everything you want, but that there are one or two things you would
like to change – so change them. Will that upset someone else?
Possibly. But it is your life that is at stake. If something is really

important to you, try to figure out a way of achieving it with minimum stress to anyone else who is involved. Remember though, if you are facing cancer, or a possible recurrence, this is no time to be putting other people first, you have probably been doing this for much of your life. This is the time to put your own life into better shape. You may even be surprised at how many positive spin-offs there are for other people when you do this.

Martine J

Martine, a wife for eight years and a mother for nearly seven, hated housework and being stuck around the house all day, but believed that she had to be there for the children and that home help was expensive. Her cancer alert was small and she responded well to treatment, but it set her thinking. Finally, she sat down with her husband and two children. She explained that she really wanted to get out more and thought she could earn enough to pay for a cleaner and, when needed, a child minder. They were surprised at her level of frustration and discontentment, but once this was understood they agreed to give her a plan to try. She did as she planned and was quickly rewarded. Her husband was happy to find she had the time and energy for him in the evenings rather than struggling with domestic chores that had carried over from the day. Her children found her more relaxed and willing to spend time playing with them or helping with their schoolwork. And as a family they spent more time enjoying themselves at the weekends. They were no better off financially, the belief that had stopped her making this move in the past, but they were all a lot happier.

If you decide that what you would have to do to achieve some of these goals is not worth the price, then recognise this and stop focusing on the lack of this goal.

Penny Y

Penny told me, during her consultation, how much she envied my ability to travel frequently, saying that was one of the things she really missed. When I pointed out that she could not travel as I had been doing, with her children, she came to recognise that she got much more pleasure out of her time with her children than she would have from being childless and having the freedom to travel, and she stopped feeling cheated by being, as she had been putting it, 'stuck at home'.

Now let's look at list five. What you would have done differently? In response to each item ask yourself:

- What did you do that you wish you had not done?
- What have you done to reverse this?
- What has stopped you?
- What could you do about it now?
- What did you not do that you could have done?
- What have you done to make up for that now?
- What can you do now to compensate for that?

You may think it is too late to change, but no, you almost certainly can, at least to some degree and in some way – possibly one that you have not yet thought of.

Perhaps you wanted to be a historian but your father insisted you learn a useful profession and become an accountant. You could still study history: go to evening classes, get a degree from the Open University or set yourself a course of study covering your favourite period. You may say, 'What's the point?' but if it now seems pointless and no longer interesting, then perhaps it is time to drop this as a regret you have been harbouring. On the other hand you might become knowledgeable about a particular type of history, even one that could relate to a niche in your present accountancy career.

One of my patients had wanted to be a cellist, but her parents had insisted she learn something useful, and so she became a librarian. After we discussed this she decided to explore the history of early cellos and then she wrote a book on it. With self-publishing a possibility, she was able to produce copies for her friends. But the main benefit was the joy she experienced as she immersed herself in the topic, exploring libraries and the Web, and meeting up with people with a similar interest.

The benefit of the exercises

The point of these mental exercises is both diagnostic and therapeutic. When you do them you will learn a lot about yourself. Dealing with them is part of your therapy. You may find you have been harbouring regrets that, in truth, you no longer feel. You may come to see that you have achieved more than you have been recognising. You may discover some accessible changes you can make to improve your life. The important thing in all of this is to increase your positive states and minimise the negative ones.

Your mind may be more powerful than you realise.

There is a much quoted study undertaken by Steven Greer and written up in the *Lancet* medical journal in 1990.[103] It is a prospective study started in 1972 involving a group of women with stage-2 breast cancer where some had spread into surrounding tissues. They were interviewed three months after their original diagnosis and could be divided into four groups:

1 **Fighting spirit** Those whose dominant reaction was 'I will fight this thing and win', and who set out to learn all they could and to do as much for themselves as they could, either as the sole treatment or to augment whatever conventional therapy they chose to have.

2 **Denial** Those who buried their heads in the sand and refused to think about it, ignored it and got on with their lives as if it didn't exist, refusing to let it depress or worry them, only hearing the positive information that they wanted to hear and blithely assuming that all would be well.

3 **Stoic acceptance** Those who accepted the diagnosis, in true British stiff-upper-lip style, but who avoided learning anything more about it. They did as they were told by their doctors without delving any further,

believing that there was nothing they themselves could do about it and that 'the establishment knows best'. They endured stubbornly, stoically and in silence without asking questions or complaining.

4 **Helpless and hopeless** Those who were overwhelmed by the situation and immediately expected the worst. They sunk into the disease, let it rule their lives. They were in a state of constant fear and anxiety, feeling like helpless victims of an unkind fate.

Greer found that 'recurrence-free survival' was significantly more common in patients who showed either 1 or 2 rather than in 3 or 4. Thirteen years after the start of the study 80 per cent of the Fighting Spirits (group 1) were still alive and well, but only 50 per cent of the Deniers (group 2), 30 per cent of the Stoics (group 3) and 20 per cent of the Hopeless and Helpless (group 4).

Many criticisms have been levied at this study, but not all of them are valid and a lot of positive use can be made of it; for example, it can be said that the Fighters don't just live longer because of their inherent positive mental state; they get better because they take positive action and adopt a number of changes that can help in their recovery. This is true, but this attitude and behaviour pattern is also a part of their positive mental state. Either way, being one of those in group 1 offers the best chance of a positive outcome. If you are not inherently in that group, then it could be worth attempting to become and act like that group.

A Positive Attitude

You are almost certainly aware of the placebo effect. If you think, or are convinced, that a medication will cure you it probably will, even if it is only water. This effect is so powerful that it has to be allowed for when testing any new drug. Your mind can heal you, if you just give it a chance. There are many dozens of books on positive mental healing. The good ones work. Read them and put the ideas into action.

I am totally opposed to people being told how long they can expect to live, whatever health problem it might relate to, but particularly if they have cancer. Such a prognosis is rarely accurate if the patient is not told. If they *are* told, however, they frequently live for just that length of time. You can think yourself well, if you think you can, and you can also do the reverse. What is important is that you harness this amazing power of your mind.

At the start you need to know that there is real substance in this perspective, so here are some simple examples. Thinking positive and optimistic thoughts changes your cellular chemistry. Try it:

1   Sit quietly and relax.

2   Think about something positive and wonderful. Let yourself smile. Do this for five minutes. Be aware of how your body feels.

3   Stop. Now think of something bad, something that makes you unhappy or stressed. Allow the frown to develop, your mouth to turn down. Do this for five minutes.

4   Feel the internal differences.

And that was just a simple imaginary exercise. Here's another:

1   Imagine a 15.25m (50ft) plank lying on the ground. Imagine yourself walking along it. Check inside and find out how your body feels.

2   Now imagine yourself at the top of a 50-storey building. Someone has put the same 50-foot plank, well supported but only from underneath, out into open space. Imagine yourself walking out along it. Check inside and find out how your body feels.

Unless you have no imagination at all, you almost certainly felt the adrenalin rushing, your palms getting sweaty and other changes occurring. This will show you how powerful your mind is.

It is important to create a positive mental attitude. This is important in prevention, it is also important if you have had cancer and are trying to avoid a recurrence. You may be able to create this positive mindset for yourself, or you may need help. Read books about people who have had cancer and who have recovered. Read about the positive benefits of the many different substances you may be taking as part of your regime. Read books on mind power. Play CDs on positive thinking. And keep doing it. Each book that you read may take you eight steps forward and then leave you to drift seven steps back, but you did gain some positive insights and move one positive step forward. Do it again, and you gain another step. Keep layering-on all this positive input. You've got nothing to lose – except your problems.

Find Supportive Groups

There is evidence that people who have, or have had, cancer and who have been part of a supportive group of people in similar situations, live longer and do better than those who try to go it alone. This works for most people. But if you truly are a loner, preferring to keep these issues to yourself, do be aware of this and do look for appropriate support in some form. You may not want to join a group, but you may need just one person who is right there, for you to talk to and unburden yourself to, as and when you need it.

Avoid negative groups. In my early years in Sydney one patient complained that she had gone to a cancer support group run by one of my colleagues and found it a totally depressing experience. Everyone, she said, was sitting around waiting to die. When I thought about it I realised that my colleague was, by Greer's classification, one of the 'helpless and hopeless' types. This meant that she was wonderfully supportive and understanding with people in distress, but perhaps more likely to see the glass half empty than the glass half full. So try to work with people who are focused on what they *can* do for you, not those that want to comfort you in regard to all the things they *can't* do for you. Avoid negative sob stories. You don't need to read about other people's bad experiences, or the failure of a particular drug or remedy. Read about the positive outcomes and remember the power of the placebo effect.

The positives

If a remedy increased the survival rate by X per cent this is good, this is what you need to focus on, not the fact that it did not achieve 100 per cent survival rates. After all, you will doubtless be doing dozens of different therapies, or taking many different remedies. Each of them will contribute to your health and well-being. They are all additive. The more you do (within reason and without conflict) the more successful you will be. Detoxing improves your chances of recovery, so does the correct diet, making good nutritional deficiencies and correcting metabolic errors. Some people have recovered totally just doing this much. More people have benefited from removing all the predisposing factors in their life. When you put your whole programme together your odds of both avoiding cancer and avoiding a recurrence are terrific. Best of all, with these huge steps in health improvement, your risk of developing all the other diseases, such as heart attacks, strokes, diabetes, arthritis and more, will diminish proportionately. You may well reach old age being much healthier than your friends who did not either get cancer or have to worry about a recurrence.

CHAPTER 20

Predisposing Factor No. 12 – Exhausting Your Adrenal Glands

We have discussed emotional stresses, but there is also physical stress. This results when you demand more of your body than it is capable of, in the long term. We can call this overload. Overload occurs when some or all of these things happen: you work long hours; you are given more to do than you can handle; you do not give yourself time for rest and relaxation; you fail to get sufficient sleep; or you generally push yourself beyond what is healthy. Overload can be made up of bad stresses when they threaten to overwhelm you. It can also include neutral or good stresses. You may insist that you love what you are doing; yes, you work hard, but you love every minute of it and do not find it stressful. Indeed, you may say that it is fulfilling and adds to your enjoyment of life; nonetheless it can still be overstressing your body. This type of stress – this pleasant overload – can sometimes be more insidious and dangerous for not being recognised as something that is potentially harmful.

So it's time now to consider how your body handles emotional stresses and physical overload and how an excess of either or both of these can be major predisposing factors for cancer. Conversely, removing the stressors and reducing the demands you make on your body can help you to reverse out of the cancer process. It is important that you understand how this works, for it is all too easy to underestimate the destructive power of this predisposing factor.

The Adrenal Glands and Stress

Your adrenal glands are a pair of glands that sit on top of your kidneys. They play a key role in the way you handle stress – both immediate and acute stress on the one hand and prolonged and chronic stress on the other. There are two parts to each of these adrenal glands: the outer part, or cortex, which produces the steroid hormones such as cortisone, cortisol, corticosterone, aldosterone, oestrogen, progesterone and testosterone, and the inner part, or medulla, which produces adrenalin and noradrenalin.

It is a significant simplification, but it is possible to consider that the medulla plays a major role in handling acute stress, in producing the burst of adrenalin that helps you deal with the sudden and acute emergencies, and that when stress is chronic and prolonged the cortex and its hormones come into play.

There is a general tendency by those in the medical profession to fail to recognise or pay adequate attention to adrenal exhaustion. It frequently underestimates or ignores the impact that adrenal exhaustion can have on general health and, conversely, it ignores the impact that poor health can have on the adrenal glands, which become even more stressed or exhausted once an illness develops. This escalating state can lead to further health problems in a self-perpetuating cycle. Whole books are written on both stress and fatigue[104] yet the care of these two glands is often ignored.

How the adrenal glands work

To understand the theory, it is necessary to understand in a little more detail how your adrenal glands work. These glands are part of your hormonal system. When you are stressed, chemically, physically or mentally, hormones, such as one called adrenocorticotropic hormone, or ACTH, travel from your brain to your two adrenal glands. These glands are then stimulated to produce and release the various hormones that they manufacture.

Several of the adrenal hormones are part of your fight-or-flight mechanism. During periods of stress the adrenal glands are stimulated, adrenalin is then produced and flows through your bloodstream. From here it acts on various cells throughout your body. Blood flow to your arms and legs is stimulated so that you can run or fight; the blood flow through your lungs and heart is increased, enabling you to deliver more oxygen to your muscles so that you can run further and faster. Conversely, the actions of your digestive processes and waste-disposal activities are stopped, as they are rightly deemed to be inappropriate at this time. This also means that the extra blood needed at the extremities can be drawn from your abdomen around your digestive system.

The phases of stress

Hans Selye, whom we met in the previous chapter, recognised the universal changes that occur when you are stressed. He also recognised that this pattern of change was fundamental to all types of stress, whether pleasurable or unpleasant, and that it underlies all illnesses and disease processes. He recognised, and delineated, three phases of stress which, put simply, are as follows:

1 **In the alarm phase** there is a sudden rush of adrenalin output. This leads to the possibility of immediate action, of coping with the crisis and of performing such feats of strength that are not normally possible. This is accomplished in many ways. The peripheral blood vessels dilate, allowing for a greater flow of oxygen and nutrients to every part of the target tissue. Some cells store glucose as part of the much larger glycogen molecule; adrenalin stimulates the breakdown of this glycogen into glucose so that it is available for the production of a quick and dramatic burst of energy.

This method of handling stress was appropriate when we were hunter-gatherers and handling the stressors required by a physical response. It is less appropriate as a way of handling the stressors inherent in an urban lifestyle; however, our physiological evolution has not caught up with this change. Back to the story.

2 **The adaptation phase** In an ideal situation the stressor would soon be removed, your body would settle back to normal and relax, more adrenalin could be produced and used to recharge your adrenal glands. However, in our twenty-first-century lifestyle, the stressor is generally not removed. The stressful job that caused a heightened level of awareness and activity for the first few days becomes one that you learn to deal with. It does not go away, but you learn to cope. This is the adaptation phase. This phase can last for a long time, it may last for many months or even years, possibly decades. During that time you adapt, your body chemistry adapts, other hormones, including cortisol, get involved and you learn to cope, both chemically and in your lifestyle. You may come to think you are invincible and that you can keep going at this level forever. You may

even become proud of the fact. Alternatively, you may recognise that it cannot go on, that you are running out of the capacity to cope, that you need a break – yet perhaps you can't take one. Eventually all your adaptive and coping capacity is used up.

3 **The exhaustion phase** is reached. At this point the same alarm is experienced as at the start: your adrenal glands receive the message to act heroically and cope with the crisis, and more adrenalin is required. But your adrenal glands are exhausted, they cannot respond; adequate amounts of adrenalin can no longer be produced. It is equivalent to lashing an exhausted pack animal. When exhaustion sets in, you are at your limit. As a result there is less oxygen available to peripheral cells, the stored glycogen builds up and cells become glycogen-engorged. Dr Waltraut Fryda,[105] in her book *Diagnosis: Cancer,* has suggested that in an effort to cope with that the cells turn to anaerobic metabolism, utilising only the EM pathway and not the Krebs cycle (explained in Chapter 16); in other words, they turn cancerous.

This makes adrenal exhaustion a very harmful predisposing factor for cancer.

Recognised and unrecognised adrenal illnesses

Medical science recognises that all other glands can be either hypoactive or hyperactive. The thyroid gland, for example, can either produce too little or too much thyroxin, and in either case ill health results. The pancreas can produce either too little or too much insulin and again, in either case, ill health can result. An excess of adrenal activity is recognised and leads to a disease called Cushing's syndrome. Acute damage to the adrenal gland leads to Addison's disease, associated with hypo function of the gland; however, and somewhat surprisingly, the medical profession does not often recognise the less dramatic, chronic, functional adrenal exhaustion and deficiency disease that can build up over time, yet it is arguably very common and can have far-reaching adverse consequences.[106]

Of itself, adrenal exhaustion is a predisposing factor that can start you along Phase One of the cancer process; however, when it is prolonged or becomes severe, it is a powerful component of Phase Two of this process as well. Failing to deal with this and resolve any stressors aggravates the condition and hinders any form of therapy.

Dr Fryda believes that adrenal exhaustion is the major and most significant predisposing factor in the development of cancer, so do not take it lightly. Do the test (below). Your glands may be more stressed than you think.

Testing for the Vital Signs

The Adrenal Stress Index is a test that you can readily organise for yourself at home, although you will generally be asked to provide the name of your practitioner when you order the test. The required kit can be obtained from one of the testing laboratories. You will generally be asked to collect four saliva samples at four stated times over a full day and evening. You collect these by spitting into a tube until there is sufficient saliva for the test to be performed. You then post the samples to the laboratory where measurements will be made of your levels of two hormones, cortisol and DHEA, hormones that are indicators of prolonged stress. The results will tell you where you are along the scale from the 'alarm phase' to the 'exhaustion phase'. DHEA is also tested for in part of the CA Profile offered by American Metabolics.

Your Optimising Strategy

If the results show you to be physiologically stressed, you should improve your diet and make good any nutrient deficiencies (see Chapters 9–12). Reduce your intake of alcohol, coffee and other non-nutrient stimulants. Using stimulants or temporary energy boosters is no way to help your adrenal glands, it only lets you drive them even harder and into ever more complete exhaustion.

Vitamins and minerals

Nearly all the vitamins have a role to play in your adrenal glands. Beta-carotene is the major carotenoid required. Vitamins B_1, B_2, B_3 and B_5 are needed for the production of energy in these glands, and additional B_5 is need for the synthesis of adrenal corticosteroid hormones; you may need as much as 500mg, even 1,000mg of this vitamin if your adrenal glands are seriously exhausted. Vitamin B_6 is needed for the conversion of the amino acid tyrosine into adrenalin. Folic acid and Vitamin B_{12} are needed for the synthesis of DNA and adrenalin. Vitamin C is present at high concentrations in the adrenal glands and is needed for steroid synthesis. It is a valuable antioxidant, and it prevents conversion of beneficial adrenalin into toxic adrenochrome and of beneficial noradrenalin into toxic noradrenochrome. Several bioflavonoids (often thought of as part of the vitamin-C complex) act as local anti-inflammatory agents and support tyrosine uptake by the adrenal glands so that it is available for conversion into these two hormones. Vitamin E is concentrated in the adrenal glands, where it acts as an antioxidant, protects adrenal hormones and reduces damaging lipid peroxidation.

Minerals are also important. Potassium is needed in generous amounts and, in addition to the high vegetable diet already recommended, you could be well advised to look for a potassium salt rather than the usual sodium salt. Potassium salt is sometimes sold as 'low sodium salt' and contains potassium chloride instead of sodium chloride. Copper is needed for a number of reactions, including the conversion of tyrosine into adrenalin (although an excessive intake of copper can be dangerous if you have cancer), magnesium is needed for energy production, and manganese, selenium and zinc as antioxidants.

A number of amino acids are important for adrenal function, including glutamine and taurine in addition to tyrosine. Other beneficial compounds include coenzyme Q_{10}, N-acetyl cysteine (NAC) and lecithin. Liquorice is a particularly important herb and should be taken two hours before each of the salivary-spit-test times for which your result was below normal.

Many nutrients are needed, and there is considerable interplay between them. What you take should be based on the results of some of the tests recommended earlier. If this does not achieve the improvement you are after, you should ask for help from your CAM practitioner.

Taking stress-reduction seriously

The other half of the optimising strategy involves reducing your stress levels as discussed in the previous chapter. Build some relaxation time into your day; even if it is only for half an hour, it could make all the difference and enable you to get things done better and faster afterwards.

Even if you claim you do not feel stressed, it is important to make sure you have not overloaded your adrenal glands, as they are a vital part of both prevention and recovery. I cannot count the number of patients I have seen who have claimed not to be stressed, but who, when tested, have turned out to be in various stages of adrenal exhaustion. So do the tests now and, if the need is indicated, do all you can to correct the situation.

If you want to stay healthy and keep out of the cancer process, it is vitally important that you reduce the stresses in your life. Remove them if you can; if not, at least work on your own personal development and change your attitude to them.

CHAPTER 21

Predisposing Factor No. 13 – Underactive Thyroid Gland

Earlier in Part Three we discussed general predisposing factors, such as diet, nutrient levels, digestion, energy production and toxins. With the discussion based on sugar metabolism and your adrenal glands in more recent chapters we have moved into more specific pathologies or problems. Another major problem may relate to the function of your thyroid gland.

Many people who develop a tumour are found to have an underactive thyroid gland and, as a result, a low metabolic rate, poor energy production and a low body temperature, which in turn impacts adversely on their immune function.[107] These have already been discussed as predisposing factors and so an underactive thyroid gland can certainly be considered to be a predisposing factor and something that has to be corrected if you are endeavouring to avoid cancer.

Maximum Body Energy Requires an Efficient Thyroid

Your energy is the product of the activity and energy output of all your cells. Put another way, for you to feel fully energetic it is important that you make sure that all your cells are operating to maximum efficiency. Providing your cells with all the correct nutrients, and supporting your adrenal glands will help your body to produce energy efficiently, but this is not the whole story. Even if your cells are willing to pump out all the energy you need, they cannot do this if they do not receive the appropriate triggers or instructions. One of these triggers comes from your thyroid gland.

Your thyroid gland is situated in your neck, each half either side of the midline in the front. When your brain receives the message that you are either too cold or are lacking in energy, it sends thyrotropin releasing hormone (TRH) from the hypothalamus in your brain to your pituitary gland, next to your brain. This gland then responds by sending thyroid-stimulating hormone (TSH) down to your thyroid gland. Your thyroid gland responds by producing and sending out thyroid hormones T3 and T4. These in turn go to the various tissues throughout your body and stimulate them into action, thus increasing their metabolic activity. Your whole metabolic rate increases and you burn food energy faster. More of it is turned into energy and less into fat, so you feel warmer and more energetic – and your cellular function is improved.

Why it's important as cancer prevention

A normal metabolic rate and a good body temperature are important in preventing cancer. For one thing, you will need the energy for defence, attack and repair; for another, your immune system functions more efficiently when your temperature is up and not lagging below the normal range. Heat is an important part of fighting a tumour. A low resting body temperature can hinder recovery. This factor is given major consideration in the Anthroposophical approach to cancer, to its prevention, and to its treatment with mistletoe extracts. Mistletoe is used to stimulate immune function and the success of this treatment is partially monitored by the way it induces both a gradual rise in body temperature and an increasing diurnal spread from the highest to the lowest reading in a day as health improves.

A number of nutrient deficiencies can be caused by hypothyroidism (abnormally low activity of the thyroid gland). For instance, if you have this condition, you will need extra vitamin A in your diet because the other source of this vitamin, beta-carotene, is only converted slowly into vitamin A if your thyroid gland is underactive. A low level of T4 reduces the absorption efficiency for vitamin B_{12}, so you will need additional amounts of this to avoid becoming deficient in it.

Testing for the Vital Signs

If you ask your doctor to provide you with a test for thyroid function he or she will suggest a blood test to measure your levels of TSH, T3 and T4;

however, the normal ranges are very wide, and it is all too easy for these tests to miss a mild but significant suboptimal thyroid function. In addition, the hormones may be being produced yet not achieving the desired response.

Self-administered temperature test

There is a much simpler test that you can do yourself, at home. It costs nothing and the only equipment you will need is a thermometer. To understand the test, think about the way you measure the effectiveness of the central heating. You do it by measuring the temperature within the rooms, not by the amount of hot water or air flowing through the system or the amount of heating fuel available for the boiler. In the same way it makes better sense to measure the efficiency of your thyroid gland by the amount of heat generated in your body, rather than by the amounts of stimulating hormones flowing through your bloodstream. In fact this is the only real way to know whether or not these stimulating hormones are being effective.

Prepare the thermometer the night before, shaking it down if it is a mercury one. On waking, place the thermometer under your armpit and remain as relaxed as possible. Read the temperature. It should be between 36.6°C and 36.8°C (97.8°F and 98.2°F). If it is below this, you need to take action to increase your thyroid function.

Your Optimising Strategy

If your results are sufficiently poor, your doctor may suggest that you take thyroxin, a thyroid hormone. If this happens you will probably be told that you will have to stay on this medication indefinitely, as there is no expectation that this will improve the production or function of your own thyroid hormones. In fact, taking hormones by mouth can make your own thyroid gland lazier. After all, your brain gets the message that there is plenty of T3 and T4 around (albeit from the pills) and so your metabolism must be fine. It may even be less encouraged to produce TRH, TSH and the thyroid hormones, and so the medication can aggravate the problem, ensuring that you really do need to be on the medication for life.

The better answer is to stimulate your thyroid system into correct function. This can be accomplished by a remedy called Thyroidea Thymus, a low-potency complex (multi-component) homoeopathic remedy produced by a company called Wala in Germany. It is generally available in the German equivalent of health-food shops, but unfortunately it has recently been withdrawn from general sale in the UK, as have many CAM remedies, even though they are safe and harmless. I have used it successfully on countless patients for several decades. You may be able to get it if you know people on the Continent, and if you can, it is well worth the effort.

Vitamins B_2, B_3, C and E will help your thyroid gland to produce the thyroid hormones. Iodine is an essential component of T3 and T4. There are three atoms of it in T3 and four in T4, hence their names. A useful source of iodine is kelp, in either powdered form or tablets. A copper or zinc deficiency can lead to a reduced level of T3. Selenium is needed for the conversion of T4 to T3. Iron deficiency can lead to hypothyroidism.

The amino acids L-carnitine, L-phenylalanine, L-tyrosine are needed for the synthesis of T3 and T4. L-phenylalanine is converted into L-tyrosine which, with iodine, makes up the T3 and T4 molecules.

A number of messages have to be passed across cell membranes for the whole sequence of reactions to work and for this it is important that the cell membranes are sufficiently fluid. This is a result that can only be achieved if you have a sufficient amount of the essential fatty acids in your diet (see Chapter 9).

In summary: normal thyroid function requires many different nutrients. If you have carried out the tests recommended earlier you will know if you are deficient in any of them, in which case you can add them as supplements. If you still cannot improve your basal resting temperature, then it is probably time to ask your practitioner for help.

CHAPTER 22

Predisposing Factor No. 14 – Poor Immune Function

Your immune system is your major active defence against foreign invaders, bacteria, viruses, moulds, worms and other pathogens. It should detect foreign organisms and substances and protect you from them. By definition, therefore, it should also protect you from cancer cells; it should recognise them as being foreign and kill them. Yet clearly, if you have cancer, your immune system has failed to do this.

However, if you do have cancer it is not entirely the fault of your immune system, as cancer cells have some very clever ways of 'hiding' from it and avoiding attack by it. Nonetheless, a healthy immune system is a vitally important part of your defence mechanism, and a weakened immune system is a predisposing factor to developing cancer. It is therefore important that you understand something about the way it works.

How Your Immune System Works

The structure and function of your immune system is complex, and the following is a highly simplified version. In essence, your immune system is composed of two parts. There is the innate immunity with which you were born, and acquired immunity that you develop as you are exposed to more and more pathogens. Alternatively, it can be divided differently into humoral (body fluids) immunity and cell-mediated immunity

1 **Humoral immunity** is based on the actions of antibodies (chemicals produced by your B-cells, or B-lymphocytes, in response to antigens or foreign or toxic agents) and the various chemicals, such as cytokines and related enzymes, that act with them. These processes are facilitated by a

variety of helper cells. The removal of the pathogens is facilitated by the complement system based on the action of a number of different protein molecules.

2 **Cell-mediated immunity** involves a wide range of cells such as natural killer (NK) cells, T-lymphocytes, macrophages, basophils, neutrophils and eosinophils (occasionally called acidophils), monocytes, leukocytes and Kupffer cells. Some of them are grouped under the term 'white blood cells', although many of these, while travelling through your blood also move out and patrol your tissues (see Glossary). Chemically, their actions are facilitated by a variety of cytokines, including interleukins and interferon. These are chemicals that are secreted by some of the various cells of your immune system and pass on messages to other cells of your immune system somewhat in the same way that hormones do.

All of these cells and chemical reactions must work efficiently for you to be healthy. If any part of the system fails, you become increasingly susceptible to ill health, diseases in general and cancer in particular. From this it is easy to see that if, for example, a nutrient deficiency makes some of your cells less active, there can be a considerable knock-on, or domino, effect throughout other aspects of your immune system.

The immune cells, phagocytes and granulocytes

Many immune cells are called phagocytes, meaning that they recognise and engulf toxins and foreign organisms such as viruses and bacteria. Others are called granulocytes, which means that they contain granules, usually filled with toxic chemicals, that they can use to kill any foreign bacteria. Some cells are markers, notifying the rest of your immune system that they have detected a problem. Some hold station, others travel. In most instances there is a degree of overlap of their various activities: phagocytes can also be granulocytes, and so on. Among them all there is a complex and extensive network of communication systems.

Keeping you protected

Your first barrier to foreign invaders is the physical one that surrounds you. It is made up of your skin and the mucous membranes lining your genitourinary tract, your digestive system and your respiratory system. Not only is this a physical barrier but it also contains large numbers of sIgA antibodies (chemicals) and scavenger cells, which help protect you from invaders. In fact, this is the major part of your immune system. Keep the invaders out and you will have little trouble inside.

A faulty or inadequate immune system is absolutely a predisposing factor for cancer. Yet many forms of chemotherapy and radiation treatment work against your immune system, the hope being that these procedures will destroy the cancer cells before they completely destroy the host, and that in the final outcome the host will survive but not the cancer cells. Unfortunately, this is a long way from certain. This means that if you have decided to have chemotherapy or radiation treatments, you should be even more thorough in the CAM therapies you apply to protect and restore your own immune function (see Your Optimising Strategy below).

Testing for the Vital Signs

There are innumerable tests that can be carried out to assess your immune function. As there are too many to list here you should discuss the various possibilities with your practitioner.

The interpretation of these tests is complex and something to be left to your practitioner, who will use them to decide on the appropriate steps for you to take to ensure optimum immune function; however, helping to maintain a healthy immune system and thus prevent many possible immune problems is well within your hands once you have been told what you, personally, need to do.

Your Optimising Strategy

Just as the activity of your immune system is complex, so are its needs.

An important step in any health problem is to rebuild your immune function, which is being stressed as a result. As it is incredibly complex, it should come as no surprise to find that it demands many nutrients if it is to work efficiently. It requires, either directly or indirectly, a full complement of all the nutrients in terms of quality and quantity, macro and micro, that your body needs. Some of these nutrients are more important than others, and the ones that are important for you personally will be indicated by the results of your tests for nutrient levels.

Proteins

You need an adequate amount of protein because a deficiency can suppress the activity of your immune system. This can be animal or fish protein, or vegetable protein, provided both the quantity and quality are adequate for your metabolic needs. Your metabolic type will influence your choices (as explained in Chapter 9).

All the amino acids, derived from proteins, are needed by your immune system. Many different amino acids are needed for the production of the many hormones, antibodies and neurotransmitters that act within your immune system. Whereas half the hormones, such as oestrogen and cortisol, are made from fats and based on the steroid nucleus that is found in cholesterol, the other half are peptide hormones, which are made from amino acids. Below are some examples that are particularly useful, and they are all amino acids that are available in supplement form from health-food shops. If you have done the ONE test referred to on page 95 you will have a list of the amino acids in which you may be deficient. A urine test for amino acids will have given you more specific information as to which ones you should supplement with, and the amounts to take.

Arginine, now generally recognised as one of the essential amino acids, as few people make it in sufficient amounts, increases the response of your T-lymphocytes to antigens and increases their anti-tumour activity. It increases your production natural killer (NK) cells.

Carnitine, a combination of two amino acids, methionine and lysine, increases your production of lymphocytes. It also helps to reduce some of the negative effect that fats have on your immune system by increasing the transport of fatty acids from your bloodstream into your cells for breakdown or utilisation.

Glutamine Your level of glutamine falls after any sort of tissue damage, and especially after burns, infections, surgery and trauma. Think of this if you have had cancer and have had surgery or radiation treatment. A glutamine deficiency can have major consequences, as not only is it needed in its own right, for repair and many other reasons, but it is also a valuable source of spare amino groups that may be needed for the synthesis of many of the amino acids that you can make within your own cells.

Taurine, an amino acid used by your liver and in the production of bile, increases the ability of neutrophils to kill bacteria and engulf other toxins.

Clearly, both your total protein intake, and the consumption of adequate amounts of the various individual amino acids are important to the health of your immune system.

Fats

Fats are important, particularly the essential fatty acids. It is important that all the various messages that fly around your immune system get through to their receiving cells. This in turn means that your cell membranes must be sufficiently flexible and receptive, hence your requirement for these essential fatty acids, both in absolute amounts and in the correct ratios of omega-3 to omega-6 to omega-9 (see Chapter 9).

The best fats to consume are those obtained from fish, particularly the oily fish (but your choice will also be based on what is best for your metabolic type), those found in flaxseeds and flaxseed oil for the protective omega-3 fatty acids, and in hemp oil for a balance of omega-3 and omega-6 fatty acids. Other useful or safe fats or oils include coconut oil, which you may recall is anti-viral, anti-bacterial and anti-fungal, among other benefits, and olive oil. Although the fats found in butter and milk are saturated, they include the short-chain and medium-chain saturated fats that help in the absorption of calcium and so, of the various animals fats, are much less of a risk than those found in meat fat.

To avoid confusion, it is important to make the following distinction. In milk, the main problem in relation to cancer seems to be casein, the milk protein, whereas butter is made with the fat from the milk. If you are concerned, then don't eat butter. If you love it, there is probably no harm in eating small amounts; ideally it should be organic and preferably from unpasteurised milk.

A high intake of animal fats can be a problem and, independent of the often-associated lack of the fibre in the diet, has been shown to increase the risk of colon cancer.[108]

Further problems can result if the fats are over heated; for example, deep-fat fried red meat has been associated with an increased risk of breast cancer.[109] Processed meats are a problem, partly due to the changes in the chemistry of the fats and partly due to the various preservatives used.[110] Overheating vegetable oils can also increase the risk of cancer. Even breathing in the fumes from overheated oils can be dangerous and has lead to an increased risk of lung cancer.[111]

In general, animal fats are high in arachidonic acid, which can increase the risk of cancer. An excess of arachidonic acid, found mainly in meats, may cause lymphoid tissue to atrophy and lead to a reduced response of your T cells to antigens.[112]

Saturated fats can reduce the flexibility and function of your cell membranes. They may even cause your thymus and lymph glands – all of which are parts of your immune system – to shrink and become less effective, and to reduce the ability of phagocytes to engulf and destroy pathogens.[113]

A deficiency of the essential fatty acids leads to an overall reduction in immune function and the atrophy of lymphoid tissues. Their absence leads to weakened structure of the membranes of the cell and the cell organelles and this, as we have seen, adversely affects cell function and cell-to-cell communication and response. Remember that it is important to have enough of the omega-3 and omega-6 essential fatty acids, and to have them in the correct proportions. Use the tests and a diet analysis to determine this (see Chapter 10).

Sugar and stimulants

Your immune system gives you another reason to avoid sugar, in all its forms. Sugar stimulates insulin output, and insulin may reduce the activity of your lymphocytes. It can also lead to reduced production of antibodies (the proteins found in the blood that react with antigens or foreign substances), to reduced warning by the immune system of the presence of antigens and to decreased phagocytosis, (engulfing solid particles by the membrane of the protective cell). In other words, eating sugar handicaps your immune system, seriously.

Don't drink coffee, it may suppress the activity of your lymphocytes and the level of your protective immunoglobulins. Fortunately, this does not apply to the therapeutic coffee used in enema solutions, which generally goes directly from your colon to your liver and rarely enters your general or systemic circulation. Alcohol in moderate amounts, possibly one to two glasses in a day at the most, and preferably red wine, may be acceptable. In excessive amounts it can reduce immune function.[114]

Vitamins

Nearly all the vitamins are needed by your immune system. A vitamin A deficiency reduces the response of T and B lymphocytes to antigens and mitogens, and of antibodies to antigens. It may also reduce the production of sIgA by the cells along the walls of your digestive tract and of phagocytes. Severe deficiency of this vitamin can lead to atrophy of your thymus gland and spleen – important components of your immune system – and can significantly reduce the number of your circulating leukocytes and lymphocytes, which are important cells of your immune system.

The carotenes, closely related to vitamin A, are antioxidants. They protect phagocytes from auto-oxidation, increase the production and function of T and B lymphocytes, increase the action of macrophages, cytotoxic T cells and NK cells against tumour cells, and increase the production of interleukins.

Deficiencies of most of the B group vitamins weakens the function of your immune system in more ways than there is space to list here.

Vitamin C The need for vitamin C during infections is well known and it may well be the first vitamin you turn to when you have a cold or some other viral infection. A lack of this vitamin can lead to a delayed response by your neutrophils, reduced phagocytosis and chemotaxis (chemotaxis can be thought of as cells following a chemical trail) and an overall delay in the response of your immune system to any challenge or danger. All of these faults can be corrected, at least in part, and insofar as they are due to a lack of vitamin C, by supplementing with the vitamin; this can also increase the production of two other sub sets of your immune system, immunoglobulins and complement.

There is nothing so easy to achieve as failure. Many people have taken small doses of vitamin C and then claimed that they did not get the expected benefit. A moderate amount, of a few grams (a few thousand milligrams), may help at the start of a cold, but if you have a bad case of flu you will need to take sufficient to get to bowel-tolerance level to achieve your goal. This means absorbing as much as you can right up to the limit of almost having diarrhoea, and continuing to 'top up' to this level to keep your tissues fully supplied.

Most foods that contain vitamin C also contain a wide range of the many hundreds of different bioflavonoids. These offer benefits of their own; they also appear to help potentiate the activity of vitamin C. For instance, the French chemist, Professor Jack Masquelier, undertook pioneering research on a subgroup of bioflavonoids called oligomeric proanthocyanidins (OPCs) found in red grape skins and seeds, and found that vitamin C became 11 times more effective when used with them than when it was used on its own.[115] You will achieve a much better result if you combine the vitamin C with a variety of bioflavonoids or use a plant-derived source, than if you take ascorbic acid, or mineral ascorbates, alone.[116]

Your first step should be to improve your diet so that you increase your intake of vitamin C and bioflavonoids from fruits, vegetables and herbs. Your next resource should be supplements, preferably those derived from a variety of natural plant sources. If you need even greater amounts, or if you choose to ask your practitioner to give it to you by intravenous injection, you can then turn to pure vitamin C (ascorbic acid).

Vitamin D helps to maintain the number and activity of your T cells.

Vitamin E is needed to maintain the response of your antibodies to antigens, and to reduce the levels of prostaglandin-2 series of compounds. You will recall from Chapter 10 that this group includes many of the (possibly inappropriate or unwanted) inflammatory cytokines.

Minerals

Also important are:

Copper A lack of copper can lead to reduced levels of cell-mediated immunity, including reduced activity of granulocytes against microbes, and this in turn can lead to the increased occurrence of infections. Copper is necessary for angiogenesis, the building of new blood vessels. This is needed for growth and repair; however, it also helps to feed a tumour.[117] For this reason, and if you have cancer, you should avoid any supplements containing copper unless tests show you to be deficient in it.

Selenium is probably the mineral most recognised as being helpful to your immune function and of particular importance in relation to cancer. A deficiency can lead to reduced cell-mediated immunity (even worse than that induced by a vitamin-E deficiency), reduced phagocytosis, reduced response, or number, of several types of your immune cells, and reduced humoral immunity. Just as an excess of copper can be harmful, an excess of selenium, probably greater than 800mcg per day can be unhelpful and, in this case, can suppress immune function.

Germanium can increase the production and activity of several of your immune cells. **Iodine** is needed by your thyroid gland and a lack of it can lead not only to hypothyroidism but also to reduced anti-microbial action by the leukocytes. **Iron** deficiency can lead to reduced activity of leukocytes, particularly neutrophils, and NK cells; however, an excessive intake of iron should be avoided, particularly if you have cancer. High levels have been found to be associated with increased risk of cancer.[118] So test thoroughly for this mineral before supplementing with it.

Magnesium A deficiency of magnesium is associated with a reduced number of antibody-producing cells, reduced humoral response to antigens, and atrophy of your thymus gland. Supplementation with **manganese**, a mineral that is often in short supply both in the diet and in supplements, can increase the activity of macrophages and NK cells.

Zinc A zinc deficiency can lead to a reduced humoral response and reduced T cell numbers and response, plus reduced thymic hormone activity. Again, too much can cause problems and, in this case, may inhibit lymphocyte and neutrophil response.

Keep in mind that the relative amounts of the various minerals are as important as the absolute amounts. Remember that if you take zinc without manganese you may make yourself (more) manganese deficient, as these two minerals compete with each other for absorption from your intestines into the bloodstream. This is yet another reason why you are encouraged (a) to do the tests to find out what you need; and (b) to consult a professional to determine how best to redress any imbalances you may have.

There are many other substances that are beneficial to your immune system and are available, either from your diet or as supplements. They include coenzyme Q_{10}, which increases the activity of macrophages;

dimethyl glycine (DMG), which increases humoral and cell-mediated immunity and the production of antibodies and lymphocytes; glucosaminoglycans, which improve antibody response; and picolinic acid, which stimulates macrophage activity and can be given as zinc picolinate or chromium picolinate, depending on which mineral you most need.

Herbs and plants

Although there are many herbs and related plants that boost immune function, some of the more important or better known are medicinal mushrooms such as reishi, shiitake, cordyceps and maitake mushrooms. Other plants include astragalus, ligusticum, schizandra and European mistletoe (*Viscum album*). Helpful herbs include silymarin, bilberry, garlic, cayenne, echinacea, aloe vera juice, suma, cat's claw (increases phagocytosis), myrrh, red clover and goldenseal.

From this you can see just how important it is that you have a full complement of all the vitamins, minerals, amino acids, and essential fatty acids that you need, and how much benefit you can derive from a range of phytonutrients or phytoactive compounds from plants, including foods and herbs. This further underlines the reasons for correcting deficiencies of any of these substances, and so reducing your predisposing factors. If you would like to learn more about this topic see M.T. Murray, *Encyclopedia of Nutritional Supplements* (1996).

For a discussion of inflammation as a predisposing factor to cancer, see Appendix page 263.

CHAPTER 23

Predisposing Factor No. 15 – Faulty Oestrogen Ratios

Oestrogen and oestrogen therapies are often, and rightly, blamed for breast cancer and for other hormone-related cancers,[119] such as endometrial, uterine and ovarian,[120] and prostate cancer.

Certainly, it has a part to play. Yet a woman's level of oestrogen decreases with age, whereas her risk of developing breast cancer increases, as the following figures from the US show.

> Age 30–39: 0.43 per cent (or 1 in 233)
> Age 40–49: 1.44 per cent (or 1 in 69)
> Age 50–59: 2.63 per cent (or 1 in 38)
> Age 60–69: 3.65 per cent (or 1 in 27)[121]

What is Oestrogen?

Oestrogen, as the word is commonly used, is a collective term, covering many different compounds with certain common features and similarities. The different forms of oestrogens depend on both their source and their chemical structure. There are phytoestrogens, or oestrogen-like compounds, which are produced by plants; mycoestrogens, or oestrogen-like compounds, produced by fungi; and other oestrogens produced by animals and humans, which differ from species to species. There are also xenoestrogens, man-made compounds that are either similar to, or mimic the actions of, oestrogen. The latter are generally produced or introduced as a result of agricultural and industrial practices and are commonly found in cosmetics and medications.

The amounts of these xenoestrogens now present in our environment, in the food chain and in cosmetics, toiletries and from other sources, is rising, and their effects are cumulative and generally harmful. Many of the xenoestrogens mimic the behaviour of human oestrogens. Others have different adverse effects. The metabolism of oestrogen can lead to the production of a number of different compounds that are excreted in your stool or urine. Some of these are carcinogenic.

In humans, there are different forms of oestrogen. They all contain the steroid nucleus, the same nucleus that is found in cholesterol, and then each one has unique side chains, or groups, attached to this nucleus. Common forms of oestrogen include oestrone, oestradiol and oestriol.

The two important types: 2-OHE1 and 16a-OHE1

There are two types that are of interest to us here: 2-hydroxyestrone (2-OHE1) and 16a-hydroxyestrone (16a-OHE1). Of these, 2-OHE1 *inhibits* the occurrence and growth of tumours, while 16a-OHE1 actually *encourages* tumour formation and growth. The ratio of 2-OHE1 to 16a-OHE1 is a guide as to your relative risk of developing breast or other oestrogen- or hormone-related cancers. Obviously, it is beneficial to have this ratio as high as possible, within the normal range.

The ratio is part of your unique metabolism, and if it is inherently low you may have an inherently higher risk than other people of developing cancer;[122] however, if it is low there are things you can do to increase it.

Testing for the Vital Signs

The ratio of 2-OHE1 to 16-OHE1 can be measured in a urine sample. When you receive the sample kit from the testing laboratory you will be told the best days to take the test in relation to your menstrual cycle, if you are still menstruating. You will also be told to limit your fluid intake for at least 12 hours beforehand so that you do not dilute the urine. In your result report you will usually be told the level of each of the two forms, and the ratio of the good (2-) form to the harmful (16-) form.

Your Optimising Strategy

If your ratio is low and there is an excess of the potentially harmful 16- form as compared to the beneficial 2- form you will want to do all you can to minimise your risk of developing an oestrogen-related cancer.

Two important supplements to consider are indolyl-3-carbinol (I-3-C)[123] and di-indolylmethane (DIM). I-3-C is converted in the acid environment of your stomach into a number of compounds one of which is DIM. DIM is particularly protective of your health and helps to balance your oestrogen forms.[124]

For the conversion of I-3-C to DIM to occur there has to be sufficient acid production in your stomach. In Chapter 13, I explained that many people, particularly as they get older, suffer from undiagnosed hypochlorhydria, or lack of adequate amounts of stomach acid (pages 135–138). This is one of the many reasons why I described deteriorating digestion as a significant predisposing factor for cancer. Sick people, of any age, are particularly prone to hypochlorhydria and as such may not convert I-3-C to DIM with any efficiency, and are therefore more susceptible to oestrogen-related cancers. If you take I-3-C in supplement form, you may also want to take a supplement containing hydrochloric acid to assist in its conversion to DIM. Alternatively, you may choose to take a supplement of DIM, although this way you may be missing out on some possible benefits of other compounds also produced from I-3-C.

Cervical cancer

Cancer of the cervix is thought to be due to human papilloma virus (HPV) and this has responded to treatment with I-3-C.[125] Better still, studies have shown that that a regular intake of I-3-C can help prevent cervical cancer.[126]

In one study, four out of eight women with cervical cancer given 200mg of I-3-C a day, and in another, four out of nine women given 400mg a day, had complete regression. This compared to women in the control groups of whom none experienced regression of their tumour.[127]

It has been shown in many studies that DIM is beneficial for a number of reasons:

- DIM has been found to be helpful in fighting other oestrogen-related cancers.[128]
- It reduces the amount of the harmful 16a-OHE1.
- It helps you to maintain high levels of 2-OHEI.
- It improves detoxification and helps the liver by stimulating enzyme production in both Detox Phase One and Detox Phase Two pathways.
- DIM inhibits the growth of cancer cells by acting at the genetic level where mutations can occur.[129]
- DIM encourages apoptosis, or voluntary cell death, of cancerous cells.

DIM can be combined with chemotherapeutic agents, such as tamoxifen, used in the medical treatment of breast cancer. This will be reassuring to you if you do develop cancer and do not wish to forsake the medical route but want to add other therapies to your treatment programme. Your practitioner will advise you.

Male Cancers

DIM has advantages for men too. Androgens are male hormones, somewhat analogous to the oestrogens in females. Androgens are important for the normal development and function of the prostate gland, but when things go wrong they are also implicated in the development of prostate cancer. In the later stages of prostate cancer the cancer cells commonly become resistant to androgens and grow independently of the hormones.

Prostate cancer is usually treated with anti-androgen drugs such as Codex. DIM is the first plant-derived chemical discovered that acts as an anti-androgen, and so it was investigated for its benefit in the prevention and treatment of prostate cancer.[130] Androgen-dependent cancer cells that were treated in the laboratory with a solution of DIM grew at only 30 per cent of the rate of untreated cancer cells. DIM had no such harmful inhibitory effect on healthy cells.

Other tests have shown that DIM inhibits the actions of DHT, the main androgen or male hormone implicated in prostate cancer, which stimulates the production of prostate specific antigen (PSA). The PSA level was found to fall when androgen-dependent cells were treated with DIM.[131]

General

In summary, DIM is thought to be effective in the prevention and treatment of a number of female cancers. It is active in the treatment of viral-related cervical cancer, and is thought to be a useful compound in the treatment of prostate cancer. It is also active against a number of other types of cancer. All of which makes it a very useful substance to include in any preventive protocol.

I-3-C occurs in a number of foods, particularly in the vegetables of the broccoli and cabbage family. There is a good correlation between a high consumption of these vegetables and a reduced risk of developing cancer, particularly oestrogen-related cancers. If you put 'broccoli cancer' into a search engine on the Internet you get nearly a quarter of a million references, and for almost every type of cancer, so overwhelming is the confirmatory evidence for this.[132]

In addition to eating broccoli you should eat sprouted broccoli seeds.[133] You can buy them, but try growing your own from seeds and having them freshly to hand. The sprouts have up to 100 times the amount of I-3-C, when compared to broccoli itself.[134] The sprouts have a strong peppery taste, and if you do not like this you can find a number of products that contain powdered sprouted broccoli together with other nutrients, such as sprouted wheat powder, tomato and beetroot powder. These make very nutritious, protective and pleasant-tasting seasonings, and are very much better than the commercial stock cubes found in the supermarkets that have a number of doubtful ingredients and are laden with salt. You can also purchase supplements of I-3-C or ready-made DIM in tablet form. We have focused on broccoli, but the whole cabbage family can offer benefits.[135]

A 400mg dose of I-3-C is roughly equal to 400g (14oz) of raw cabbage or Brussels sprouts, or about 225g (8oz) of broccoli, and this produces approximately 40mg of DIM. This means that to get 200mg of DIM from eating broccoli you would have to eat about 1.25kg (2½lb) of raw broccoli. This is a large task, but it is made easier if you juice the broccoli or eat the sprouted seeds. It is also easier to get at least some of your DIM as a supplement.

Prevention being better than cure, you should avoid sources of xenoe-strogens and animal and plant oestrogens, which can trigger or increase the risk of oestrogen-related cancers. This will generally mean eliminating all cosmetics and toiletries based on petrochemicals and other chemical additives and replacing them with ones derived purely from natural plant sources, ideally organically grown and produced. Dr Hauschka and Weleda brands are good examples of these. Make sure that all your meat and dairy products are organic, to reduce your intake of farm-added hormones.

CHAPTER 24

In a Nutshell

You may have read through the whole book or dipped into those chapters that seemed particularly relevant to you. I hope that you have felt empowered by what you have read and that you feel you have a clear idea of the ways you can help to protect yourself from the cancer process by being better informed and changing your diet and lifestyle. In this chapter I give you a summary of the key points that I have made, to give you an overview of the ground we have covered.

Cancer is not simply a tumour. The tumour that is generally accepted as the evidence of the existence of a cancer is, in fact, the end product of a long and usually symptomless process of cellular changes. It is the final, detectable, symptom of these changes.

Cancer is a process, one I have called 'the cancer process'. It starts with small errors of metabolism with little significance and progresses to ever more serious problems until cells turn from healthy cells into permanent cancer cells.

There are two phases to this cancer process. In Phase One you do not have cancer, but as your errors of diet and lifestyle accumulate through the years you are progressively increasing your likelihood of developing cancer. This phase starts some significant time before a tumour is formed. Given the errors that can occur from birth onwards, it could even be said that this process, moving the body away from perfection, starts soon after birth. In Phase Two you have crossed the threshold. Up to this point, any cancer cells that you develop have been destroyed by the normal processes of your body's defence and repair mechanism. From this point onwards, these cancer cells are resistant to destruction and start to increase in number until eventually there are sufficient of them to constitute a detectable tumour.

Destroying the tumour does not stop the cancer process. Getting rid of the tumour does not stop the process any more than getting rid of the visible part of a weed destroys the network of underground roots. This is one of the reasons why so much of the medical approach is so often unsuccessful. Removing the tumour, be it with a knife, radiation or toxic chemicals, does not halt or reverse the cancer process.

Cancer occupies a tissue or organ but is not a failure of that tissue or organ. Breast cancer is not a failure of breast function, nor is colon cancer a failure of colon function, although it may lead to it. So, although we are dealing with a process that has lead to a tumour in a particular organ or tissue, the successful treatment is not going to be based on correcting or supporting the function of that specific organ or tissue.

Cancer is a systemic problem. Phase Two of the cancer process involves systemic changes that occur throughout your body. Only by recognising these and correcting them can you overcome cancer in the long term. These changes include such things as lowered pH, reduced supply of oxygen to the cells, the presence of toxins, in the widest meaning of the word, and nutrient deficiencies.

Identified risk factors increase your risk of cancer. Risk factors are the recognised factors that are associated with an increased risk of cancer. Firstly, these are generally based on a recognition of the association, often based on relative statistics. Examples include a history of HPV overgrowth and cervical cancer, and cigarette smoking and lung cancer. Then an explanation is proposed or a mechanism is elucidated. Yet there are anomalies with this. After all, not all smokers develop cancer, nor do all women with HPV. Nonetheless, if you are wise you will avoid the risk factors as far as possible; however, many of them may have already occurred in your past, such as exposure to asbestos or radiation, or a history of cigarette smoking or heavy alcohol consumption. There is little you can do to change these. There are others that you cannot change, such as your age or the number of children you have had.

Predisposing factors increase your risk of cancer. Predisposing factors may be dangers that are less obvious to you than the more publicised risk factors, but may also be a lot more potent. Unlike risk factors, predisposing factors are all part of your lifestyle and the present state of your body and health. They may not be generally recognised as risk factors, yet they greatly increase your risk of developing cancer. They are all things you can change or reduce once you recognise them.

Vital Signs can warn you of the presence of predisposing factors. You can test for these errors or problems. You can test for what I have called the Vital Signs that will warn you of your risk of developing a range of degenerative diseases up to and including cancer. When you have identified these Vital Signs and the predisposing factors they indicate, you can then set about correcting the various errors in both your diet and lifestyle on the one hand and your health on the other.

You can assess some Vital Signs for yourself. We have covered a number of Vital Signs and tests that you can do for yourself. You can determine your metabolic type and correct your diet. You can measure your pH with a simple strip of pH paper. You can check for an overgrowth of *Candida albicans* by spitting into a glass of water first thing in the morning. You can check at least some of the nutrient deficiencies in your diet. This immediately gives you the power to start reversing out of the cancer process (Phases One or Two) and doing something positive for yourself.

You will need the help of a practitioner. This is a self-help book, but it is not a do-it-yourself book. Cancer is a serious business and you will need the help of a practitioner if you truly want to be sure that you are doing all you can for your health. Some of the test results will have come with a report that includes indications regarding helpful supplements. In general you can select the vitamins, minerals and other supplements that have been indicated. But for practical reasons you will need a practitioner to request many of the tests for you. They will then be available to help you in the interpretation of your results and in the implementation of corrective or optimising procedures. I hope that the information provided in this book will inform you as to the type of help such a practitioner should be able to give you and so help you to choose your practitioner wisely.

Many Vital Signs are detected by laboratory procedures. Although you can do some of the tests and much of the basic assessment, you will certainly need the help of a number of laboratories to do the majority of the tests. Such laboratories are listed in the Appendices and many of them will provide you with information, even if you need a practitioner to actually authorise the tests you require.

Correct the predisposing factors. If you want to reverse out of the cancer process, as far as you possibly can, you will need to do all you can to remove as much or as many of the identified predisposing factors as you can. Your practitioner will guide you in this, but the ultimate day-to-day discipline that is required to do it will be up to you. By keeping in mind the explanations given here it should be easier to recognise the benefits of making these positive changes and so easier to stick to them.

You are in control. Since the great majority of cancers are caused by diet and lifestyle, arguably up to 90 per cent, by removing your predisposing factors and following this strategy, you can significantly reduce your risk of developing cancer or of having a recurrence, if you have already had cancer. The exciting and positive aspect of this is that this understanding of the cancer process, and all that is entailed, empowers you – it enables you to take control of your health and your future. If you do not do this you will be, like so many people, simply living day to day and blindly hoping that a disease that affects approximately 40 per cent of the population will somehow pass you by. The odds are not good. They can be improved enormously if you take control and act on the information given here.

There is always room for improvement. No matter how good you think you diet is, or your lifestyle, you cannot be sure that all is well. Many patients have come to me with minor problems only to find, when tested, that there were serious problems brewing, problems that, as yet, did not produce any obvious overt symptoms. The only way to know the true state of your health is to do the various tests outlined above.

The CA Profile. In my view, everyone would benefit from doing the CA Profile test (see pages 55–6). If it is clear, you can be relatively sure that you have not entered into Phase Two of the cancer process. If it is not clear you will have received an early warning sign, possibly a very early warning sign, that can help you to correct your health before the pre-cancerous or early cancerous cells have turned into a significant tumour.

Your journey to improving your health starts today. Take the tests, implement the optimising strategies, minimise your predisposing factors and reduce your risk of developing cancer or of having a recurrence.

APPENDICES

Inflammation as a Predisposing Factor for Cancer

One topic that merits further attention is the role of inflammation in the cancer process. It was highlighted at a conference called Confronting Cancer as a Chronic Disease: Primary Care Takes a 360 Degree View in May 2010 on nutrition and cancer hosted by the Institute of Functional Medicine. Many now recognise that chronic inflammation can lead to, or aggravate cancer, or its recurrence.[136]

Inflammation can be acute such as the immediate response to a wound or local infection, and it can be chronic. Acute inflammation is a short-lived change in the local chemistry, appropriate to the current challenge, and is not generally a predisposing factor for cancer. Chronic inflammation is a predisposing factor and the longer the condition persists the greater is the risk.[137]

Inflammation has many different causes including viruses, bacteria, moulds, other parasites, chemical agents and irritants, and foods to which you may be allergic or sensitive.

Examples of inflammation-induced or associated cancers include:

- Epstein-Barr virus (EBV) increases the risk of B-cell non-Hodgkin's lymphoma.
- Inhaled irritants, such as asbestos and other airborne particulates increases the risk of mesothelioma and lung cancer.[138,139]
- Reflux oesophagitis increases the risk of oesophageal cancer.[140]
- *Helicobacter pylori* bacterial infection may double or treble the risk of stomach cancer.[141,142,143]
- HIV increases the risk of non-Hodgkin's lymphoma, squamous cell carcinomas, and Kaposi's sarcoma.[144]
- Hepatitis B or C[145] or alcohol-induced inflammation, increases the risk of liver cancer.[146]

- Gall bladder inflammation and greater bile output increases the risk of colon cancer (this can be reduced by the use of a drug that reduces bile output).[147]

- Irritable (inflammatory) bowel disease, ulcerative colitis or Crohn's disease increase the risk of colon cancer five to seven-fold, often preceded by benign polyps.[148]

- Pelvic inflammatory disease increases the risk of ovarian cancer[149] and other gynaecological cancers.[150]

- Human papilloma virus (HPV) increases the risk of cervical cancer.[151]

- Many chemical carcinogens cause oxidative stress and inflammation.[152,153,154]

Some of the above cancers are clearly related to inflammation; others, such as those caused by some viruses, may be due solely to the viral-induced changes within the cells, but it is thought that there may also be an inflammatory process involved.

How Does Inflammation Lead to Cancer?

White blood cells increase in number and concentrate at inflammatory sites. They produce compounds such as arachidonic acid (otherwise known as omega-9 fatty acid, which is also found in meats), the precursor to the prostaglandin PGE2 series, cytokines and free radicals which lead, over time, to the production of mutagens.

Cells can die by apoptosis or necrosis. In apoptosis faulty cells commit suicide; phagocytes recognise this and absorb most of the breakdown products, thus limiting the damage to surrounding tissues and avoiding inflammation.[155] Necrotic tissue breakdown follows external insults. Cells die before this is recognised by the phagocytes and so the debris is released, dispersed and can lead to inflammation[156] and possible tumourigenesis.[157]

Inflammation is accompanied by the need for tissue repair and a new blood supply, thus angiogenesis is increased[158] helping to provide a blood supply both for wound healing and for any mutated cells.[159]

Testing for the Vital Signs

C-reactive protein (CRP) is raised in chronic inflammation in response to increased levels of Interleukin-6. Your erythrocyte sedimentation rate (ESR), the rate at which your red blood cells precipitate when your blood is allowed to stand, may increase indicating inflammation. Most laboratories will do both of these tests.

Many other tests can assess the state of your immune system and the possibility of inflammation. The entire topic is complex and you should consult your practitioner to explore this further.

Your Optimising Strategy

Eat lots of fresh vegetables and fruit.[160] Oxidative stress is associated with inflammation and many of the phytonutrients in these foods are antioxidants and so can help to reduce the risk of inflammation. Cancer cells themselves may produce many oxidising agents[161] and induce inflammation, hence the benefit of antioxidants.

Several proteolytic enzymes have been found to reduce chronic inflammation, including bromelain[162,163,164] derived from the stem of the pineapple and papain[165] derived from papaya. Papain has helped to reduce athletics-induced inflammation.[166] Serrapeptase is a rapidly-acting anti-inflammatory[167,168] derived from an enterobacteria originally detected in silkworms.

Non-steroidal anti-inflammatory drugs (NSAID), such as aspirin, reduce the production of inflammatory compounds; however they provide an increased risk of developing stomach ulcers and related problems which in themselves can cause further problems. Do not take NSAIDS, the enzymes plus essential fatty (omega-3) acids are better.

Glossary

Acetyl choline A neurotransmitter that also performs other functions.

Acidophils More commonly called eosinophils, a type of white blood cell.

ACTH Adrenocorticotrophic hormone, produced by the brain and acts on the adrenal glands.

Adipose tissue Fatty tissue where lipids are stored, mainly as triglycerides.

Adrenalin A hormone produced by the medulla (centre) of your adrenal glands. It is produced in response to stress and a fall in blood glucose level. It also acts as a neurotransmitter.

Aerobic Oxygen rich.

Amino acids Small compounds containing a few carbon atoms, plus at least one amino (nitrogenous) group and one acid group. They are constituents of protein but also play roles in the body as individual compounds.

Amylase A starch-splitting enzyme found in the saliva and produced by the pancreas that catalyses the breakdown of amylose.

Amylopectin A form of starch.

Amylose A form of starch.

Anaerobic Without oxygen.

Angiogenesis The process of building a new blood supply.

Antibodies Chemicals produced by B-cells in response to antigens.

Antigens Foreign or toxic substances, perceived by your immune system to be harmful. In auto-immune diseases this antigen may be a part of your own body.

Apoptosis Voluntary suicide, as occurs in old or faulty cells.

ADP Adenosine diphosphate, lower-energy molecules.

ATP Adenosine triphosphate, high-energy molecules.

Arterioles Small blood vessels, smaller than arteries, that carry oxygenated blood to the tissues.

Avidin A compound found in raw egg whites, but destroyed by heat. It combines with biotin in the digestive tract and thus prevents the absorption of the biotin. Biotin is an essential nutrient, made by intestinal bacteria. Thus eating raw egg whites can create a biotin deficiency.

Basophils A type of white blood cell.

BBB Blood–brain barrier. This is not a structural barrier in the sense of a skin around the brain. Rather it is a chemical barrier that keeps unwanted substances out of the individual cells that make up the brain.

B-cells B-lymphocytes. Cells of your immune system which produce antibodies.

BSL Blood sugar level. A measure of the amount of glucose circulating in your bloodstream.

CA 125 A cancer marker for ovarian cancer.

CA 15-3 A cancer marker for breast cancer.

CAM therapy Complementary, Alternative and Metabolic therapy. This is somewhat analogous to naturopathy.

Capillaries The very fine blood vessels that carry the blood through the tissues and from which nutrients can flow out into the tissues, and waste products and other compounds can enter the blood to be carried away by the venules.

Carboxypeptidase A protein-splitting enzyme produced by the pancreas.

CEA Cancer embryonic antigen.

Cell membrane Cell wall, consisting of a lipid–lipid bilayer with embedded proteins.

Chelating agent Chelaten = claw. An agent that combines with other molecules, usually mineral atoms.

Choriocarcinoma A type of cancer that occurs during pregnancy if embryo growth does not slow down.

Chymotryspin A protein-splitting enzyme produced by the pancreas.

Corpus luteum A temporary endocrine structure that produces progesterone.

Cytosol The matrix of the cell within which the various cell organelles and structures are located.

DGLA Dihomo-gamma-linolenic acid.

DHA Docosahexaenoic acid.

DHEA Dehydroepiandrosterone.

Differentiated cells Fully matured cells that have developed the appropriate specialised characteristics of the tissues of which they are a part. These cells have lost their ability to subdivide or multiply.

Disaccharides Molecules made up of two single monosaccharides joined together. Examples include sucrose, maltose and lactose.

DNA Deoxyribonucleic acid, made up from your genes.

DMPS 2, 3-Dimercapto-1-propanesulfonic acid, a chelating agent.

DMSA Dimercaptosuccinic acid, a chelating agent.

Dopamine A neurotransmitter.

EDTA Ethylenediaminetetra acetic acid – a chelating agent.

EGFR Epidermal growth factor receptors that increase glucose uptake by cancer cells.

EM pathway Embden–Meyerhof pathway. The anaerobic pathway that occurs in the cell's cytoplasm and converts glucose to either lactic acid or pyruvic acid.

Endocrine system Your hormone system.

Enzymes Biological catalysts. Their name usually ends in —ase and the start of the word provides information as to the compounds involved in the reaction or the type of reaction.

EPA Eicosapontaenoic acid.

Epithelial tissue Tissue made up of the cells that line the cavities and surfaces of the body.

FIR Far infrared.

Fibroblasts Cells that produce the fibres which hold connective tissues together.

FOS Fructo-oligosaccharide. A prebiotic that helps beneficial bacteria such as *Lactobacillus acidophilus* and other probiotics become firmly established in your digestive tract.

Free radicals Highly active and dangerous 'bits' of molecules, unlike ions and far more active, generally destructively so.

Geographic tongue A tongue that is not smooth and uniform but has irregular patches of varying colour or textures, possibly with fissures.

GABA Gamma aminobutyric acid, a neurotransmitter.

GLA Gamma linolenic acid.

Glands Specialised tissues that produce hormones. Examples include the thyroid and adrenal glands.

Glycemic index An indication of the extent to which a food increases your blood glucose level. A food with a high-glycemic index raises your blood glucose level higher than one with a low-glycemic index.

Glycogen The large macromolecule composed of glucose units synthesised in the liver and muscles. Sometimes called 'animal starch'.

Glycogenolysis The breakdown of glycogen into glucose.

Glycolysis The breakdown of glucose via the Embden–Meyerhoff pathway in the cytosol of the cell.

Glycoprotein A molecule with a carbohydrate (such as glucose or fructose) and a protein part (or an amino acid group).

GTF Glucose tolerance factor, contains chromium and vitamin B_3 and helps insulin to trigger cellular uptake of glucose from the bloodstream.

HbA1C A combination of glucose and haemoglobin, often raised in the blood of people with diabetes.

HCG Human chorionic gonadotropin. The hormone produced by early embryonic cells and cancer cells.

Hydrophillic Water-loving, or water-attracting, substances that can dissolve in water.

Hydrophobic Water-hating or water-repelling, substances that are generally more soluble in lipids (fats).

Hypochlorhydria Lack of hydrochloric acid production in the stomach.

ITP Insulin potentiation therapy.

Krebs cycle The sequence of reactions in the mitochondria that releases approximately 95 per cent of the energy from carbohydrates and lipids.

Lipids Fats and oils, composed mainly (but not only) of fatty acids, substances that are 'oily' or 'greasy' to the touch.

Metastasis The development of secondary malignant growths at a distance from the primary site of cancer.

MDS Medical–drug–surgery.

Micron A unit of length. One millionth of a metre.

Mitochondria Organelles within cells in which components of carbohydrates, fats and proteins are oxidised with the release of energy, carbon dioxide and water.

Mitogen A substance that triggers cell division.

mmol/l A unit to measure concentration, such as the amount of glucose in 1 litre (1¾ pints) of blood.

Monosaccharides Single sugars. Examples include glucose, fructose, galactose and ribose.

Morula A cluster of cells at the earliest stage of embryonic development.

Mucous membranes line body cavities, not all of them secrete mucus.

Naturopath Someone who functions rather like a general practitioner but who follows the naturopathic philosophy and uses natural remedies instead of medical drugs.

Naturopathy Definitions vary, but as used in Australia, where I trained, it was the umbrella term for nutrition, herbal medicine, homoeopathy and an extensive range of other natural therapies. It does not generally include chiropractic, osteopathy or Eastern medical disciplines.

Neurotransmitter A chemical messenger molecule produced by and sent out by nerve cells.

Neutrophils A type of white blood cell.

Noradrenalin A hormone produced, like adrenalin, in the adrenal medulla but also elsewhere in the body. A neurotransmitter.

Nutriceuticals Analogous to pharmaceuticals but made up of beneficial nutrients.

Oestrogen A group of several different hormones relating to female sexual characteristics and activities, produced by the female ovaries and the adrenal cortex (outer layer) in both sexes.

Oligosaccharide Several single sugar units, up to about eleven, such as glucose, joined together.

Organs Specialised structures within the body such as the liver, kidneys or heart.

PDGF Platelet-derived growth factor, a hormone that stimulates angiogenesis.

Peptides Chains of amino acids, very much smaller than proteins.

Peristaltic action The muscular movement of the walls of your digestive tract that moves the food and food residues along.

Peroxisomes Cell organelles involved in fatty acid catabolism; contain the enzymes needed to break down toxic peroxides, produced mainly during lipid catabolism.

Phagocytosis The act of a cell engulfing a foreign particle or object.

Phytonutrients Nutrients found in plants.

Prebiotics Substances, such as FOS, that help probiotics to establish and flourish.

Predisposing factors Risk factors, nutrient deficiencies, toxins and a wide range of health problems, some major, some seemingly minor, that increase your risk of developing cancer.

Probiotics Beneficial mircoorganisms. Usually applied to those that inhabit your digestive tract.

Progesterone A female hormone produced in varying amounts throughout the menstrual cycle.

Prostaglandins Compounds derived from fatty acids that can be thought of as micro hormones. They act locally.

PSA Prostate specific antigen.

PSNS Parasympathetic nervous system. This deals with your internal housekeeping, promotes the flow of digestive enzymes, peristalsis (movement) along the digestive tract, the preparation and expulsion of waste solids and of urine. Blood is pooled in your abdomen for nutrient absorption. This system can only operate when your SNS (sympathetic nervous system) is turned off.

Receptor site An area of cell membrane, usually a protein embedded in the fatty membrane, that accepts messenger molecules arriving in the blood and passes on this 'message' to the inside of the cell. The protein may also form a channel through which compounds can enter or leave the cell.

RNA Ribonucleic acid – derived from DNA and made up from your genes.

Seratonin A neurotransmitter.

sIgA Secretory immunoglobulin A. Released by the walls of your mucosal membranes, such as those lining your intestinal system and genito-urinary tract, a vital part of your immune defence against ingested pathogens.

SNS Sympathetic nervous system. This deals with fight or flight. Blood flows from your abdomen to your limbs, lungs and eyes, so that you are ready to deal with physical dangers. It is the normal stress response even though in modern society most stressors are mental rather than physical. When this system is active your PSNS (parasympathetic nervous system) cannot function.

Totipotent cells Undifferentiated cells that still have the potential to become any cell type throughout the body.

Trans-fatty acids Normal unsaturated fatty acids are in the healthy cis form. During processing of vegetable oils and cooking of many fats the structure is rearranged into the trans form which gives rise to a number of dangerous toxins.

Trophoblast The outer layer of cells of the morula (or developing embryo).

Trypsin Protein-splitting enzyme produced by the pancreas.

Tumorlysis toxicity Toxicity due to the compounds being released when a tumour is broken down.

Undifferentiated cells Cells that still have the potential to develop into a range of cell types. These cells are capable of subdividing and multiplying.

VEGF Vascular endothelial growth factor, stimulates angiogenesis.

Venules Small blood vessels, smaller than veins, that carry deoxygenated blood from the capillaries to the veins and so back to the lungs.

Xenobiotics Substances that are foreign to your body and that should not be there.

The Cells of Your Immune System and What They Do

Basophils (granulocytes). The least common granulocytes. Present in the blood. They enter tissues when there is disease.

Dendritic cells (phagocytes) stay put and monitor their location. They enlist the help of T cells by taking hold of antigens and offering them up to the T cells. This action triggers the activity of the T cells (see lymphocytes).

Eosinophils (granulocytes). Acid-loving immune cells found mainly in the blood. They enter certain tissues only when there is disease.

Kupffer cells (phagocytes) are macrophages occurring in large numbers found along the lining of your digestive tract, in your connective tissues, lungs, spleen and along some of the blood vessels in your liver.

Leukocytes (some are granulocytes) are white blood cells, of which there are five types: neutrophils, eosinophils, basophils, lymphocytes and monocytes.

Lymphocytes are common within the lymphatic system. They include T-lymphocytes, also called T cells, B lymphocytes, also called B cells and natural killer, or NK, cells.

Macrophages (phagocytes) are found in tissues throughout the body. They secrete monokines (types of cytokines).

Mast cells are similar to basophils except that they stay in specific tissues, not in the blood. Responsible for the allergic reactions in places such as the lungs and skin.

Monocytes (phagocytes) travel in your blood.

Neutrophils (phagocytes and granulocytes) both travel in the blood and move out into the tissues.

Plasma cell A programmed B lymphocyte.

References

1 S.D. Levitt and S.J. Dubner, *Superfreakonomics*, Allen Lane (2009)

2 S.D. Levitt and S.J. Dubner, *Superfreakonomics*, Allen Lane (2009)

3 G. Morgan, R. Ward and M. Barton, 'The contribution of cytotoxic chemotherapy to 5-year survival in adult malignancies', *Journal of Clinical Oncology* (December 2004);16(8):549–60

4 Pier Mario Biava, *Cancer and the Search for Lost Meaning*, North Atlantic Books (2009)

5 A. Jemal, et al., 'Cancer statistics', *CA Cancer Journal for Clinicians* (2006); 56:106–130

6 Figures from Cancer Research UK. http://info.cancerresearchuk.org/cancerstats/incidence/?a=5441

7 Published online in the *Journal of Clinical Oncology*, picked up by CancerActive newsletter

8 S.D. Levitt and S.J. Dubner, *Superfreakonomics*, Allen Lane (2009), p. 84

9 R. Moss, *Questioning Chemotherapy*, Equinox (2004), Chapter 6, 'Toxicity of Chemotherapy'

10 *Medical Oncology* (1994);11:21–5

11 *J Gynecol Obstet Bio Repro*, (1955);24:9–12

12 A.B. Kunnumakkara, et al., 'Curcumin sensitizes human colorectal cancer xenografts in nude mice to gamma-radiation by targeting nuclear factor-kappaB-regulated gene products', *Clinical Cancer Research*, (2008)14:2128–36

13 G.L. Patrick, *An Introduction to Medical Chemistry*, Oxford Press (2009)

14 Cancer Research UK

15 See http://singularityhub.com/2009/10/12/new-cancer-detector-chip-works-in-about-30-minutes/

16 http://www.caprofile.net/

17 http://www.caprofile.net/

18 Mohammad Athar, et al., 'Resveratrol: A review of preclinical studies for human cancer prevention', *Toxicology and Applied Pharmacology*, (November 2007);224: 274–83

19 Merethe Kumle, et al., 'Use of oral contraceptives and breast cancer risk', *Norwegian-Swedish Women's Lifestyle and Health Cohort Study*

Cancer Epidemiology, Biomarkers & Prevention, (2002);11: 1375–81

20 T. Shao and Y. Yang, 'Cholecystectomy and the risk of colorectal cancer', *American Journal of Gastroenterology* (August 2005); 100(8):1813–20

21 P.J. D'Adamo, *Eat Right for Your Type,* Penguin (2003)

22 T. Campbell, et al., *The China Study: Startling Implications for Diet, Weight Loss, and Long-Term Health,* BenBella Books (2004)

23 http://www.healingdaily.com/conditions/saliva-ph-test.htm

24 http://www.healingdaily.com/conditions/saliva-ph-test.htm; H.Aihara, *Acid and Alkali,* Ohsawa Macrobiotic Foundation (1986)

25 http://www.healingdaily.com/conditions/saliva-ph-test.htm

26 See Herman Aihara, *Acid and Alkali* (1986); R.O. Young and S. Redford Young, Chapter 5 'Understanding the acid/alkaline picture', *Sick and Tired?,* Woodland Publishing (2001)

27 X.K. Williams, *What's in My Food?,* Nature and Health Books (1988)

28 Udo Erasmus, *Fats that Heal and Fats that Kill,* Alive Books (1993); Robert Andrew Brown, *Omega Six The Devil's Fat: Why Excess Omega 6 and a Lack of Omega 3 Promotes CHD, Aggression, Depression, ADHD, Obesity, Poor Sleep, PCOS, Breast Cancer, Infertility, Arthritis, and Western Illness,* Les Creux (2008)

29 Dr J. Budwig, *Cancer, the Problem and the Solution,* Nexus (2005); *The Oil and Protein Diet Cookbook,* Apple Publishing (1952); *Flax Oil as a True Aid Against Arthritis, Heart Infarction, Cancer and Other Diseases,* Apple Publishing (1994)

30 Chih V. Dang, 'A unique glucose-dependent apoptotic pathway induced by c-Myc', *Proceedings of the National Academy of Sciences* (1998);95:1511–16); 'Does sugar feed cancer?' University of Utah Health Sciences (18 August 2009) http://www.sciencedaily.com/releases/2009/08/090817184539.htm

31 R.J. Williams and D.K. Kalita, *A Physician's Handbook of Orthomolecular Medicine,* Pergamon Press (1977), Chapter 2

32 R. Moss, *Antioxidants against Cancer,* Equinox Press (2000)

33 http://news.bbc.co.uk/1/hi/health/7540822.stm; Sebastian J. Padayatty, et al., 'Intravenously administered vitamin C as cancer therapy: three cases', *Canadian Medical Association Journal* (28 March 2006); 174(7): 93–42; A. Hoffer, *Vitamin C Cancer, Discovery, Recovery, Controversy*; E. Cameron and L. Pauling, *Cancer and vitamin C: A discussion of the nature, causes, prevention and treatment of cancer with special reference to the value of Vitamin C,* Camino (1993)

34 J.M. Lappe, et al., 'Vitamin D and calcium supplementation reduces cancer risk: Results of a randomized trial', *American Journal of Clinical Nutrition*, (June 2007);85(6):1586–91

35 http://www.ars.usda.gov/Services/docs.htm?docid=18877

36 X. Williams, *What's in My Food?*, Prism Press (1988)

37 L.C Clark, et al., 'Decreased incidence of prostate cancer with selenium supplementation: Results of a double-blind cancer prevention trial', *British Journal of Urology* (1998)61:730–4; I.P. Clement, 'Lessons from basic research in selenium and cancer prevention', *Journal of Nutrition* (1998);128(11):1845–54; H.E. Ganther, 'Selenium metabolism, selenoproteins and mechanisms of cancer prevention: Complexities with thioredoxin reductase', *Carcinogenesis* (1999); 20(9):1657–66

38 A.S. Prasad and O. Kucuk, 'Zinc in cancer prevention', *Cancer and Metastasis Reviews* (2002);21(3--4):291–4

39 Y. Xu, et al., 'Mutations in the prooter reveal a cause for the reduced expression of the human manganese superoxide dismutase gene in cancer cells, *Oncogene* (1999);18(1): 93–102

40 S.Y. Yu, et al., 'Regional variation of cancer mortality incidence and its relation to selenium levels in China', *Biological Trace Element Research*, 1985;7:21–9

41 H.B. Xue, et al., 'The binding of heavy metals to algal surfaces', *Water Research* (1988);22: 917; AB Ahner, K.S. Kong, et al., 'Phytochelatin production in marine algae: An interspecies comparison', *Limnol Oceanograph* (1995);40: 649–57; H.P. Carr, et al., 'Characterization of the cadmium-binding capacity of Chlorella vulgaris', *Bulletin of Environmental and Contamination Toxicology* (1998);60(3): 433–40; M. Tsezos, 'Biosorption of radioactive species', in B.Volesky (ed.), *Biosorption of Heavy Metals*, CRC Press (1990), pp. 45–50; D. Klinghardt, 'Amalgam/mercury detox as a treatment for chronic viral, bacterial, and fungal illnesses', *Explore!* (1997);8(3)

42 X. Williams, *Overcoming Candida*, Vega (2002); M.T. Murray, *Chronic Candidiasis*, Prima (1997) http://www.candidafree.co.uk/

43 R. Kulacz and T. Levy, *The Roots of Disease*, Xlibris (2002)

44 W. Kelley, *Cancer: Curing the Incurable Disease*, New Century (2005)

45 M.M. Walker, L. Teare and C. McNulty, 'Gastric cancer and Helicobacter pylori: The bug, the host or the environment?'

Postgraduate Medicine, 84:169–70 doi:10.1136/pgmj.2008.068346 (2008)

46 M. Jarosz, et al., 'Effects of high dose vitamin C treatment on Helicobacter pylori infection and total vitamin C concentration in gastric juice', *European Journal of Cancer Prevention*, Dec. 1988; 7(6):449–54; Zun Wu Zhan and Michael J.G. Farthing, 'The roles of vitamin C in Helicobacter pylori associated gastric carcinogenesis', *Chinese Journal of Digestive Diseases*, May 2005; 6(2):53–8(6)

47 Figures from Cancer Research UK, for 2006

48 http://www.news.harvard.edu/gazette/2002/08.22/01-oral-cancer.html

49 A.W. Maksymiuk, et al., *American Journal of Medicine* (30 October 1984);77(4D):20-7; G. Bodey, et al., 'Fungal infections in cancer patients: An international autopsy survey', *European Journal of Clinical Microbiology and Infectious Diseases* (February 1992);11(2):99–109

50 X. Williams, *Overcoming Candida*, Vega (2002); M.T. Murray, *Chronic Candidiasis*, Prima (1997) http://www.candidafree.co.uk/

51 If you wish to read more, see X. Williams, *Liver Detox Plan*, Vermilion (1998)

52 P.G. Alley and S.P. Lee, 'The increased risk of proximal colonic cancer after cholecystectomy', *Diseases of the Colon and Rectum* (1983);26(8):522–4

53 X. Williams, *Liver Detox Plan*, Vermilion (1998)

54 D.J. Liska, 'The Detoxification Enzyme System', *Alternative Medicine Review* (1998);3(3):187–98

55 J.M. Berg, J.L. Tymoczko, and L. Stryer, *Biochemistry* (5th Edn), W.H. Freeman & Co. Ltd (2002)

56 Jan M. M. Walboomers, et al., 'Human papilloma virus is a necessary cause of invasive cervical cancer worldwide', *Journal of Pathology* (1999);189:12-19

57 US Department of Health and Human Studies, FDA http://www.fda.gov/Food/FoodSafety/FoodContaminantsAdulteration/ChemicalContaminants/Benzene/ucm055815.htm

58 W. Lijinsky, 'N-nitrosamines as environmental Carcinogens', Chapter 10 of Jean-Pierre Anselme (ed.), *N-nitrosamines* (1979) p. 101

59 *Explore*, March 2006;2(2):122

60 P.A. Demers, et al., 'Occupational exposure to electromagnetic fields and breast cancer in men', *American Journal of Epidemiology*

(1991);134(4):340–7; T. Tynes, et al., 'Incidence of cancer in Norwegian workers potentially exposed to electromagnetic fields', *American Journal of Epidemiology* (1992);136(1):81–8; T. Tynes, 'Electromagnetic fields and male breast cancer', *Biomedicine and Pharmacotherapy* (1993);47(10):425–7

61 K. Hemminki, et al., 'DNA adducts, mutations and cancer', *Regulatory Toxicology and Pharmacology* (December 2000); 32(3):264–75; R.M. Santella, et al., 'DNA adducts, DNA repair genotype/phenotype and cancer risk', *Mutation Research* (December 2005);30;592(1–2):29-35; L.J. Marnett and A.B. Hancock Jr., 'Lipid peroxidation-DNA damage by malondialdehyde', *Mutation Research* (Mar 1999);8;424(1-2):83–95

62 A. Brenner, 'Trace mineral levels in hyperactive children responding to the Feingold diet', *Journal of Pediatrics* (June 1979);94(6):944–5; K.R. Nolan, 'Copper Toxicity Syndrome', *Journal of Orthomolecular Psychiatry* (1983);12(4):270

63 A.G. Mainous, III, et al., 'Iron, lipids, and risk of cancer in the Framingham offspring cohort', *American Journal of Epidemiology* (2005);161(12):1115–22; A.G. Mainous III, et al., 'Dietary iron and cancer: Discussion', *Annals of Family Medicine* (2005);3(2):131–7

64 Ralf Kleef, et al., 'Fever, Cancer Incidence and Spontaneous Remissions', *NeuroImmunoModulation* (2001);9:55–64; http:// content.karger.com/ProdukteDB/produkte.asp?Doi=49008

65 G.M. Hahn, *Hyperthermia and Cancer*, Plenum Press (1982); F. K. Storm, et al., 'Hyperthermia therapy for human neoplasms: Thermal death time', *Cancer* (1975);46(8):1849–54

66 E.J. Hall and L. Roizin-Towle, 'Biological effects of heat', *Cancer Research* (1984);44:4708s–13s

67 E. Ahonen, et al., 'Fluid balance and the sauna', *Duodecim Medical Publications Duodecim* (1988);104(8):609–14

68 N. Ise, et al., 'Effect of far-infrared radiation on forearm skin blood flow', *Annals of Physiological Anthropology* (January 1987);6(1):31–2; T. Kihara, et al.,. 'Repeated sauna treatment improves vascular endothelial and cardiac function in patients with chronic heart failure', *Journal of the American College of Cardiology* (6 March 2002);39:754–9; 16:35. T. Kihara, et al., 'Sauna therapy decreases cardiac arrhythmias in patients with chronic heart failure', *American Heart Association*, Scientific Sessions (November 2002):17-20

69 D.J. Czarnowski, et al., 'Excretion of nitrogen compounds in sweat

during sauna', *Polski Tygodnik Lekarski* (18 February–4 Mar 1991);46(8–10):186–7; J.R. Cohn and E.A. Emmett, 'The excretion of trace metals in human sweat', *Annals of Clinical and Laboratory Science* (1978);8(4):270–4; Z.R. Gard and E.J. Brown, 'History of sauna/hyperthermia: Past and present efficacy in detoxification', *Townsend Letter for Doctors* (June 1992):470–8, (July 1992):650–60, (October 1992):846–54, (August–September 1999):76-86

70 I.S. Cherniaevm, 'Investigation of the permeability of human skin to infrared radiation', *Gigiena Sanitariia* (December 1965);30(12):20–4

71 E. Ernst, et al., 'Regular sauna bathing and the incidence of common colds', *Annals of Medicine* (1990);22(4):225–7

72 L. Didierjean, et al., 'Biologically active interleukin in human eccrine sweat: Site dependent variations in alpha/beta ratios and stress-induced increased excretion', *Cytokine* (November 1990);2(6):438–46

73 K. Kukkonen-Harjula, and K. Kauppinen, 'How the sauna affects the endocrine system', *Annals of Clinical Research*, (1998);20(4):262–6

74 K. Honda and S. Inoue, 'Sleep-inducing effects of far infared radiation in rats', *International Journal of Biometeorology* (June 1988); 32(2)02-4

75 *Hospital Practice* (August 1999):128, quoted by Dr N. Gonzalez www.dr-gonzalez.com/clinical_pearls.htm

76 Luke K. T. Lam, et al., 'Isolation and identification of kahweol palmitate and cafestol palmitate as active constituents of green coffee beans that enhance glutathione s-transferase activity in the mouse', *Cancer Research* (1 April 1982);42:1193–8

77 O. Warburg, 'On the origin of cancer cells', *Science* (February 1956);123:309–14; K. Garber, 'Energy boost: The Warburg Effect returns in a new theory of cancer', *Journal of the National Cancer Institute* (2004);96(24):1805–6

78 R. A. Anderson, et al., 'Elevated intakes of supplemental chromium improve glucose and insulin variables in individuals with type 2 diabetes', *Journal of the American Diabetes Association* (1997); 46(11):1786; R.A. Anderson, 'Chromium, glucose tolerance and diabetes', *Biological Trace Element Research* (1992);32:19–24 Springer; R.A. Anderson, 'Chromium in the prevention and control of diabetes', *Diabetes & Metabolism* (February 2000);26(1):22–7

79 M. Hiromura, et al., 'Glucose lowering activity by oral administration of bis(allixinato)oxidovanadium(IV) complex in streptozotocin-induced diabetic mice and gene expression profiling in their skeletal

muscles', *Metallomics* (2009);1:92; S.P. Smith, 'Trace Mineral Vanadium Against Diabetes?', *EzineArticles.com* (22 March 2008, 8 March 2010)

80 S.S. Coughlin, et al., 'Diabetes mellitus as a predictor of cancer mortality in a large cohort of US adults', *American Journal of Epidemiology* (2004)159:1160–7; M. Mazen Jamal, et al., 'Diabetes as a risk factor for gastrointestinal cancer among American veterans', *World Journal of Gastroenterology* (November 2009) 14;15(42):5274–8

81 R.J. Shaw, 'Glucose metabolism and cancer', *Current Opinion in Cell Biology, Cell division, growth and death / Cell differentiation* (December 2006);18(6):598–608; M. L. Macheda, et al., 'Molecular and cellular regulation of glucose transporter (GLUT) proteins in cancer', *Cellular Physiology* (2005);202(3):654–62; M.A. Moore, et al., 'Implications of the hyperinsulinaemia-diabetes-cancer link for preventive efforts', *European Journal of Cancer Prevention* (April 1998); 7(2):89–107

82 http://www.library.nhs.uk/diabetes/viewResource.aspx?resID= 261624

83 M. Kunitz, 'Crystalline soybean trypsin inhibitor', *Journal of General Physiology* (1947);30:291–310; R.L. Lyman and S. Lepkovsky, 'The effect of raw soybean meal and trypsin inhibitor diets on pancreatic enzyme secretion in the rat', *Journal of Nutrition* (1957);62(2):269

84 P. Quillin with N. Quillin, *Beating Cancer with Nutrition*, Nutrition Times Press (2001) p. 64; M. Rothkopf, 'Fuel utilisation in neoplastic disease: Implications for the use of nutritional support in cancer patients', *Nutrition* (July–August 1990)supp; 6(4):14S-16S

85 S. Seely, D.F. Horrobin, 'Diet and breast cancer: The possible connection with sugar consumption', *Medical Hypothesis* (July 1983);11(3):319–27

86 G.E. Demetrakopoulos, *Cancer Research* (February 1982);42:756S

87 http://www.nsc24.com/CancerR.htm

88 V. Papa, et al., 'Elevated insulin receptor content in human breast cancer', *Journal of Clinical Investigation* (1990);86(5):1503–10; Quillin, above, p. 65

89 G.E. Demetrakopoulos, *Cancer Research* (February 1982);42:756S

90 D.S. Michaud, et al., 'A diet high in glycemic load may increase the risk of pancreatic cancer in women who already have an underlying degree of insulin resistance', *Journal of the National Cancer Institute* (2002); 94(17):1293–1300

91 http://www.eurekalert.org/pub_releases/2008-05/uotm-ure050208.php

92 A. Bagust, et al., 'The projected health care burden of Type 2 diabetes in the UK from 2000 to 2060', *Diabetic Medicine* (2002);19(4):1-5; L. Haines, et al., 'Rising incidence of Type 2 diabetes in children in the UK', *Diabetes Care* (May 2007);30(5):1097–1101

93 A. Sanchez, *American Journal of Clinical Nutrition* (November 1973);26:1180–4

94 D. Yam, 'Insulin-cancer relationships: Possible dietary implication', *Medical Hypotheses* (June 1992);38(2):111–7

95 E. Simon, et al., 'Blockade of insulin secretion by mannoheptulose', *Israel Journal of Medical Sciences* (1972);8:743–52; J. Ferrer, et al., 'Signals derived from glucose metabolism are required for glucose regulation of pancreatic isletGLUT2 mRNA and protein', *Diabetes* (1993);42:1273–80; M. Board, 'High Km glucose-phosphorylating (glucokinase) activities in a range of tumor cell lines and inhibition of rates of tumor growth by the specific enzyme inhibitor manno-heptulose', *Cancer Research* (1995);55:3278–85; L. Z. Xu, et al., 'Sugar specificity of human b-cell glucokinase: Correlation of molecular models with kinetic measurements, *Journal of Biochemistry* (1995);34:6083–92.

96 C. Pert, *Molecules of Emotion*, Pocket Books (1999)

97 H. Lai, et al., 'Targeted treatment of cancer with artemesinin and artemesinin-tagged iron-carrying compounds', *Expert Opinion on Therapeutic Targets* (2005);9(5):995–1007

98 H. J. Baltrusch, et. al., 'Stress, cancer and immunity: New developments in biopsychosocial and psychoneuroimmunologic research', *Acta Neurologica* (August 1991);13(4):315–27; Lawrence LeShan, *Cancer as a Turning Point*, Plume Penguin (1994); Waltraut Fryda, *Diagnosis: Cancer*, Xlibris (2006)

99 See X. Williams, *From Stress to Success*, Thorsons (2001); L. LeShan, *Cancer as a Turning Point*, Plume (1994)

100 See also L. LeShan, *Cancer as a Turning Point*, Plume (1994)

101 I. Grigg, *EFT in Your Pocket*, New Vision Media (2005)

102 Dr K. Kermani, *Autogenic Training*, Souvenir Press (1996)

103 S. Greer, et al., 'Psychological Response to Breast Cancer and 15-year Outcome', *Lancet* (1990);335(8680):49–50

104 X. Williams, *Fatigue: The Secret of Getting Your Energy Back*, William Heinemann (1996) and *From Stress to Success*, Thorsons (2001);

L. Wilson and Jonathan V. Wright, *Adrenal Fatigue: The 21st Century Stress Syndrome*, Smart (2002)

105 W. Fryda, *Diagnosis: Cancer*, Xlibris (2006)

106 J. E. Bower, et al., 'Fatigue and proinflammatory cytokine activity in breast cancer survivors', *Psychosomatic Medicine* (2002);64:604–11; J. E. Bower, et al., 'Diurnal cortisol rhythm and fatigue in breast cancer survivors', *Psychoneuroendocrinology* (January 2005); 30(1):92–100; J. L. Ryan et al., 'Mechanisms of cancer-related fatigue', *Oncologist* (May 2007);12(supp. 1):22–34; A.J. Plechner, 'An innovative cancer therapy that saves animals: Can it help humans as well? – Cortisol Imbalances', *Townsend Letter for Doctors and Patients* (February–March 2004)

107 J. Diamond and W. L. Cowden with B. Goldberg, *Alternative Medicine, Definitive Guide to Cancer*, Future Medicine Publishing (1997) pp.383, 619; B.O. Barnes and L. Galton, *Hypothyroidism, the Unsuspected Illness* (1976); S. Venturi and M. Venturi, 'Iodide, thyroid and stomach carcinogenesis: Evolutionary story of a primitive antioxidant?', *European Journal of Endocrinology* (1999);140: 371–2; A. Tsuchiya, et al., 'Breast cancer concurrent with hyperthyroidism: A case report', *Surgery Today* (March 1981);11(2); J.G.C. Spencer, 'The influence of the thyroid in malignant disease', *British Journal of Cancer* (September 1954);8(3): 393–411

108 E. Giovannucci, et al., 'Intake of fat, meat, and fiber in relation to risk of colon cancer in men', *Cancer Research* (May 1994);54:2390–7

109 Qi Dai, et al., 'Consumption of animal foods, cooking methods, and risk of breast cancer epidemiology', *Biomarkers and Prevention* (September 2002);11:801

110 A.J. Cross and R. Sinha, 'Meat-related mutagens/carcinogens in the etiology of colorectal cancer', *Environmental and Molecular Mutagenesis* (2004);4(1);44-55

111 Tai-An Chianga, et al., 'Mutagenicity and polycyclic aromatic hydrocarbon content of fumes from heated cooking oils produced in Taiwan', *Mutation Research/Fundamental and Molecular Mechanisms of Mutagenesis* (28 November 1997); 381(2):157–61

112 J. Ghosh and C.E. Myers, 'Arachidonic acid stimulates prostate cancer cell growth: Critical role of 5-Lipoxygenase', *Biochemical and Biophysical Research Communications* (18 June 1997);235(2):418–23; Sung H. Hong, et al., 'Relationship of arachidonic acid metabolizing enzyme expression in epithelial cancer cell lines to the growth effect

of selective biochemical inhibitors', *Cancer Research* (1 May 1999);59:2223–8; M. D. Brown, et al., 'Promotion of prostatic metastatic migration towards human bone marrow stoma by omega 6 and its inhibition by omega 3 PUFAs', *British Journal of Cancer* (2006);94:842–53; J. P. Neoptolemos, et al., 'Arachidonic acid and docosahexaenoic acid are increased in human colorectal cancer', *Gut* (March 1991);32(3):278–81

113 W.J. Morrow, et al., 'Dietary fat and immune function. I. Antibody responses, lymphocyte and accessory cell function in (NZB x NZW)F1 mice', *Journal of Immunology* (1985);135(6):3857–63

114 Robert T. Cook, 'Alcohol abuse, alcoholism, and damage to the immune system: A review', *Alcoholism: Clinical and Experimental Research* (2008);22(9):1927–42

115 J. Masquelier and B. Schwittiers, *OPC in Practice*, Alpha Omega (1993)

116 J. Masquelier and B. Schwittiers, *OPC in Practice*, Alpha Omega (1995)

117 Frans J. Kok1, et al., 'Serum copper and zinc and the risk of death from cancer and cardiovascular disease', *American Journal of Epidemiology* (1988);128(2):352–9; I. Yücel, et al., 'Serum copper and zinc levels and copper/zinc ratio in patients with breast cancer', *Biological Trace Element Research* (January 1994); 40(1)

118 R.G. Stevens, et al., 'Body iron stores and the risk of cancer', *New England Journal of Medicine* (20 October 1988);319(16):1047–52; R.L. Nelson, 'Iron and colorectal cancer risk: Human studies', *Nutrition Reviews* (2001);59(5):140–8; P. Knekt, et al., 'Body iron stores and risk of cancer', *International Journal of Cancer* (2006);56(3):379–82

119 C. Schairer, et al., 'Menopausal estrogen and estrogen–progestin replacement therapy and breast cancer risk', *JAMA* (2000);283:485–91; L. Bergkvist, et al., 'The risk of breast cancer after estrogen and estrogen–progestin replacement', *New England Journal of Medicine* (3 August 1989);321(5):293–297

120 H.K. Ziel and W.D. Finkle, 'Increased risk of endometrial carcinoma among users of conjugated estrogens', *The Challenge of Epidemiology: Issues and Selected Readings*, Pan American Health Organization (1988), pp. 578–83(6)

121 National Cancer Institute, US National Institutes of Health, Fact sheet, 'Probability of Breast Cancer in Women', www.cancer.gov

122 A.O. Mueck, H. Seeger and D. Wallwiener, 'Impact of hormone replacement therapy on endogenous estradiol metabolism in post-menopausal women', *Maturitas* (25 October 2002);43(2):87–93; G.C. Kabat, et al., 'Estrogen metabolism and breast cancer', *Epidemiology* (January 2006);17(1):80–8; W.A. Olsen, et al., 'Urinary hydroxyestrogens and breast cancer risk among postmenopausal women: A prospective study', *Cancer Epidemiol Biomarkers and Prevention* (September 2005);14(9):2137–42; P. Muti, et al., 'Urinary estrogen metabolites and prostate cancer: A case-control studying the United States', *Cancer Causes Control* (December 2002);13(10): 947–55

123 K.J. Auborn, et al., 'Indole-3-carbinol is a negative regulator of estrogen', *American Society for Nutritional Sciences Journal of Nutrition* (July 2003);133:2470S–5S, Supplement: 'Nutritional genomics and proteomics in cancer prevention'

124 Chibo Hong, et al., 'Bcl-2 family-mediated apoptotic effects of 3,3′-diindolylmethane (DIM) in human breast cancer cells', *Biochemical Pharmacology* (15 March 2002);63(6):1085–97

125 Da-Zhi Chen, et al., 'Indole-3-carbinol and diindolylmethane induce apoptosis of human cervical cancer cells and in murine HPV16-transgenic preneoplastic cervical epithelium,' *Journal of Nutrition* (2001);131:3294–302

126 Liang Jin, et al., 'Indole-3-carbinol prevents cervical cancer in human papilloma virus type 16 (HPV16) transgenic mice1', *Cancer Research* (August 1999);59:3991–7; Da-Zhi Chen, et al., 'Indole-3-carbinol and diindolylmethane induce apoptosis of human cervical cancer cells and in murine hpv16-transgenic preneoplastic cervical epithelium', *Journal of Nutrition* (2001);131:3294302

127 http://lpi.oregonstate.edu/infocenter/phytochemicals/i3c

128 H. Leong, et al., 'Cytostatic effects of 3,3'-diindolylmethane in human endometrial cancer cells result from an estrogen receptor-mediated increase in transforming growth factor-α expression', *Carcinogenesis* (November 2001);22(11):1809–17; J.J. Michnovicz, 'Increased estrogen 2-hydroxylation in obese women using oral indole-3-carbinol', *International Journal of Obesity and Related Metabolic Disorders* (1998);22(3):227–9

129 F. H. Sarkar and Li Yiwei, 'Significance of indole-3-carbinol and its metabolite in human cancers', *Evidence-Based Integrative Medicine* (2003);1(1):33–41

130 Y. Li, et al., 'Gene expression profiles of i3c- and dim-treated pc3 human prostate cancer cells determined by cDNA microarray analysis', *American Society for Nutritional Sciences Journal of Nutrition* (April 2003);133:1011–9; M. Nachshon-Kedmi, et al., 'Indole-3-carbinol and 3,3'-diindolylmethane induce apoptosis in human prostate cancer cells', *Food and Chemical Toxicology* (June 2003);41(6):745–52

131 http://www.vrp.com/articles.aspx?ProdID=art1090&zTYPE=2

132 Y. Zhang, et al., 'A major inducer of anticarcinogenic protective enzymes from broccoli: Isolation and elucidation of structure', *Proceedings of the National Academy of Sciences of the United States* (15 March 1992); 89(6):2399–2403; J. Lin, et al., 'Glutathione trans-ferase null genotype, broccoli, and lower prevalence of colorectal adenomas', *Cancer Epidemiology, Biomarkers & Prevention* (August 1998);7:647; T.K. Smith, et al., 'Effects of brassica vegetable juice on the induction of apoptosis and aberrant crypt vivo', *Carcinogenesis* (2003); 24(3):491–5

133 T.A. Shapiro, et al., 'Chemoprotective glucosinolates and isothio-cyanates of broccoli sprouts metabolism and excretion in humans', *Cancer Epidemiology, Biomarkers & Prevention* (May 2001);10:501

134 Jed W. Fahey, et al., 'Broccoli sprouts: An exceptionally rich source of inducers of enzymes that protect against chemical carcinogens', *Proceedings of the National Academy of Sciences* (16 September 1997);94(19):10367–72

135 G. von Poppel, et al., 'Brassica vegetables and cancer prevention: Epidemiology and mechanisms', *Advances in Experimental Medicine and Biology* (1999);472: 159–68; 'A typical cabbage con-tains about 1,200 mg of I3C', http://www.netwellness.org/question.cfm/28063.htm

136 E. Schacter, S.A. Weitzman, 'Chronic Inflammation and Cancer', *Oncology* (2002); 16(2):217–32

137 P.M. Choi, M.P. Zelig, 'Similarity of colorectal cancer in Crohn's dis-ease and ulcerative colitis: Implications for carcinogenesis and prevention', *Gut* (1994); 35:950–54

138 K. Steenland, L. Stayner, 'Silica, asbestos, man-made mineral fibers, and cancer', *Cancer Causes Control* (1997); 8:491–503

139 K. A. Peebles et al., 'Inflammation and lung carcinogenesis: applying findings in prevention and treatment', *Expert Review of Anticancer Therapy* (October 2007); 7(10):1405–21

140 M. Pera, V.F. Trastek, P.C. Pairolero et al., 'Barrett's disease: Pathophysiology of metaplasia and adenocarcinoma', *The Annals of Thoracic Surgery*, (1993);56:1191–97

141 P. Correa, 'Helicobacter pylori as a pathogen and carcinogen', *Journey of Physiology and Pharmacology*, (1997); 48(suppl 4):19–24

142 P. Correa, 'Helicobacter pylori and gastric carcinogenesis', *The American Journal of Surgical Pathology*, (1995); 19:S37–43

143 J. Parsonnet, 'Bacterial infection as a cause of cancer', *Environmental Health Perspectives*, (1995);103(suppl 8):263–68

144 J. J. Goedert, 'The epidemiology of acquired immunodeficiency syndrome malignancies', *Seminars in Oncology*, (2000); 27:390–401

145 P. H. Hayashi, J. B. Zeldis, 'Molecular biology of viral hepatitis and hepatocellular carcinoma', *Comprehensive Therapy*, (1993);19:188–196

146 H. K. Seitz, G. Poschl, U. A. Simanowski, 'Alcohol and cancer', *Recent Developments in Alcoholism*, (1998);14:67–95

147 B. Y. Tung, M. J. Emond, R. C. Haggitt et al., 'Ursodiol use is associated with lower prevalence of colonic neoplasia in patients with ulcerative colitis and primary sclerosing cholangitis', *Annals of Internal Medicine*, (2001); 134:89–95

148 A. Ekbom, C. Helmick, M. Zack, et al., 'Ulcerative colitis and colorectal cancer. A population-based study', The *New England Journal of Medicine*, (1990); 323:1228–233

149 H. A. Risch, G. R. Howe, 'Pelvic inflammatory disease and the risk of epithelial ovarian cancer', *Cancer Epidemiol Biomarkers Preview*, (1995); 4:447–51

150 B. Goswami, M. Rajappa, M. Sharma, A. Sharma, 'Inflammation: its role and interplay in the development of cancer, with special focus on gynecological malignancies', *International Journal of Gynecological Cancer* (18 October 2007. Epub ahead of print)

151 J. Bornstein, M. A. Rahat, H. Abramovici, 'Etiology of cervical cancer: Current concepts', *Obstetrical Gynecological Survey*, (1995); 50:146–54

152 K. Frenkel, L. Wei, H. Wei, '7,12-Dimethylbenz[a]anthracene induces oxidative DNA modification in vivo', *Free Radical Biology & Medicine*, (1995); 19:373–80

153 C. A. Elmets, M. Athar, K. A. Tubesing et al., 'Susceptibility to the biological effects of polyaromatic hydrocarbons is influenced by genes of the major histocompatibility complex', *Proceedings of the National Academy of Sciences USA*, (1998); 95:14915–19

154 G.P. Casale, Z. Cheng, J. Liu et al., 'Profiles of cytokine mRNAs in the

skin and lymph nodes of SENCAR mice treated epicutaneously with dibenzo[a,l]pyrene or dimethylbenz[a]anthracene reveal a direct correlation between carcinogen-induced contact hypersensitivity and epidermal hyperplasia', *Molecular Carcinogenesis* (2000); 27:125–40

155 E. Shacter, J. A. Williams, R, M, Hinson et al., 'Oxidative stress interferes with cancer chemotherapy: Inhibition of lymphoma cell apoptosis and phagocytosis', *Blood* (2000); 96:307–13

156 J. Savill, V. Fadok, 'Corpse clearance defines the meaning of cell death', *Nature* (2000); 407:784–88

157 K. Frenkel, K. Chrzan, 'Radiation-like modification of DNA and H2O2 formation by activated polymorphonuclear leukocytes (PMNs)', in P. Cerutti, O. F. Nygaard, M. Simic (eds), *Anticarcinogenesis and Radiation Protection*, Plenum Publishing Corp (1987), pp. 97–102

158 J. R. Jackson, M. P. Seed, C. H. Kircher, et al., 'The codependence of angiogenesis and chronic inflammation', *FASEB Journal* (1997); 11:457–465

159 J. R. Jackson, M. P. Seed, C. H. Kircher et al., 'The codependence of angiogenesis and chronic inflammation', *FASEB Journal* (1997); 11:457–65

160 J. B. Blumberg, 'Considerations of the scientific substantiation for antioxidant vitamins and beta-carotene in disease prevention', *American Journal of Clinical Nutrition* (1995); 62:1521S-1526S

161 E. Schacter, S. A. Weitzman, 'Chronic Inflammation and Cancer', *Oncology* (2002);16(2):217–32

162 L. P. Hale, P. K. Greer, C. T. Trinh and M. R. Gottfried, 'Treatment with oral bromelain decreases colonic inflammation in the IL-10-deficient murine model of inflammatory bowel disease', *Clinical Immunology*; 116(2):135–142

163 K. Neetu et al., 'Regulation of p53, nuclear factor κB and cyclooxygenase-2 expression by bromelain through targeting mitogen-activated protein kinase pathway in mouse skin', *Toxicology and Applied Pharmacology*; 226(1):30–37

164 R. C. Hou, Y. S. Chen, J. R. Huang, K. C. Jeng, 'Cross-linked bromelain inhibits lipopolysaccharide-induced cytokine production involving cellular signaling suppression in rats', *Journal of Agricultural and Food Chemistry*, (22 March 2006);54(6):2193–8

165 B. Rose, C. Herder, H. Löffler, G. Meierhoff, N. C. Schloot, M. Walz, S. Martin, 'Dose-dependent induction of IL-6 by plant-derived

proteases in vitro', *Clinical and Experimental Immunology*, (January 2006);143(1):85–92

166 H. T. Holt, 'Carica papaya as ancillary therapy for athletic injuries', *Current Therapeutic Research*, (1969); 11(10):621

167 A. Mazzone, M. Catalani, M. Costanzo, A. Drusian, A. Mandoli, S. Russo, E. Guarini, G. Vesperini, 'Evaluation of Serratia peptidase in acute or chronic inflammation of otorhinolaryngology pathology: a multicentre, double-blind, randomized trial versus placebo', *Journal of International Medical Research*, (September-October 1990); 18(5):379–88

168 A. Panagariya, A. K. Sharma, 'A preliminary trial of serratiopeptidase in patients with carpal tunnel syndrome', *Journal of Association of Physicians of India*, (December 1999); 47(12):1170–2

Resources

Associations and support groups

Anthroposophic Health and Social Care provides addresses throughout the country. Includes mistletoe therapy. www.ahasc.org.uk

Anthroposophical Medical Association Raphael Medical Centre, Hildenborough Independent Hospital, Hollanden Park, Cold Harbour Lane, Hildenborough, Tonbridge, Kent TN11 9LE. Tel: 01732 833924, email: reception@raphaelmedicalcentre.co.uk

British Naturopathic Association 1 Green Lane Avenue, Street, Somerset, BA16 0QS. Tel: 01458 840072, email: admin@naturopaths.org.uk

CancerActive The Elms, Radclive Road, Gawcott, Bucks, MK18 4JB. Tel: 01280 821 211, email: enquiries@canceractive.com

Gerson Group UK PO Box 406, Esher, Surrey KT10 9UL. The helpline operates seven days a week on: 01372 464557, www.gersonsupportgroup.org.uk

Penny Brohn Cancer Care Chapel Pill Lane, Pill, Bristol, BS20 0HH. Helpline tel: 0845 1232310, www.pennybrohncancercare.org

Yes to Life Unit 7 Block C, Imperial Works, Perren St, London, NW5 3ED. Tel: 0845 257 6950, www.yestolife.org.uk

Books

Food and food preparation

Mike Anderson, *Healing Cancer from Inside Out*, Ravediet.com (2009)

Mike Anderson, *Rave Diet and Lifestyle*, Ravediet.com (2009)

Elizabeth Baker, *The Gourmet UnCook Book – The Elegance of Raw Food*, Promotion Publications (1996)

Richard Beliveau and Denis Gingras, *Foods to Fight Cancer*, Dorling Kindersley (2007)

Brian Clement, *Hippocrates LifeForce*, Healthy Living Publications (2007)

Jennifer Cornbleet, *Raw Food Made Easy*, Book Publishing Co (2005)

Gabriel Cousens, *Conscious Eating*, North Atlantic Books (2000)

Gabriel Cousens, *Rainbow Green Live-Food Cuisine*, North Atlantic Books (2003)

Jane Grigson, *Jane Grigson's Vegetable Book*, Penguin (1998)

Juliano with Erika Lenkert, *Raw, the Uncook Book: New Vegetarian Food for Life*, HarperCollins (2003)

Viana La Place, *Verdura: Vegetables, Italian Style*, Grub Street (2010)

Deborah Madison, *The Savoury Way*, Bantam (1990)

Deborah Madison, *The Greens Cook Book: Extraordinary Vegetarian Cuisine*, Grub Street (2010)

Julie Sahni, *Classic Indian Vegetarian Cooking*, Grub Street (2003)

Naomi Shannon, *The Raw Gourmet*, Alive Books (2007)

Diana Store (ed.), *Raw Food Works*, Raw Superfoods (2009)

Ann Wigmore and Dennis Weaver, *The Hippocrates Diet and Health Program*, Avery (2000)

Ann Wigmore, *Wheatgrass Book*, Avery (1987)

Kate Wood, *Eat Smart, Eat Raw: Detox Recipes for a High Energy Diet*, Grub Street (2002)

The mind and emotions

David Feinstein, Donna Eden and Gary Craig, *The Healing Power of EFT and Energy Psychology*, Piatkus (2005)

Isy Grigg, *EFT in Your Pocket*, New Vision Media (2005)

Lawrence LeShan, *Cancer as a Turning Point*, Plume (1994)

Lawrence LeShan, *How to Meditate: A Guide to Self-discovery*, Boston: Little Brown (1974)

Barbel Mohr, *The Cosmic Ordering Service: A Guide to Realising Your Dreams*, Hodder Mobius (2006)

Andreas Moritz, *Cancer is not a Disease – It's a Survival Mechanism*, Wellness Press (2005)

Dermot O'Connor, *The Healing Code: One Man's Amazing Journey Back to Health and His Proven Five-Step Plan to Recovery*, Hodder Mobius (2006)

Martin L. Rossman, *Fighting Cancer from Within*, Henry Holt and Co. (2003)

Robert Schwartz, *Courageous Souls: Do We Plan Our Life Challenges Before Birth?*, Whispering Winds Press (2006)

Xandria Williams, *Choosing Health Intentionally*, Simon Schuster (1990)

Xandria Williams, *From Stress to Success*, Thorsons (2001)

Dental work and toxins

Dr Paula Baillie-Hamilton, *Toxic Overload: A Doctor's Plan for Combating Illnesses Caused by Chemicals in Our Foods, Our Homes, and Our Medicine Cabinet*, Avery (2005)

Paul Blanc, *How Everyday Products Make People Sick*, UC Press (2007)

Russell Blaylock, *Excitotoxins: The Taste that Kills*, Health Press (1997)

Rachel Carson, *Silent Spring*, Penguin (1962)

Theo Colborn, et al., *Our Stolen Future*, Plume (1997)

Wendy Duyker, *Detox Your Home, Body and Mind*, BAS Publishing (2005)

Randall Fitzgerald, *Hundred Year Lie: How to Protect Yourself from Chemicals*, Plume (2006)

Gary Ginsberg and Brian Toal, *What's Toxic, What's Not*, Berkeley Publishing Group (2006)

Hal A. Huggins, *It's All in Your Head: The Link Between Mercury Amalgams and Illness*, Avery (1993)

Robert Kulacz and Thomas Levy, *The Roots of Disease*, Xlibris (2002)

Felicity Lawrence, *Not on the Label*, Penguin (2004)

George E. Meinig, *The Root Canal Cover-Up*, Price-Pottenger Nutrition Foundation (1997)

Michael Rutledge, *Product of Misinformation: Demistifying Cosmetics and Personal Care Claims, Terms and Ingredients*, Tapestry Press (2001)

David Steinman and Samuel Epstein, *The Safe Shoppers Bible – Consumer's Guide to Nontoxic Household Products, Cosmetics and Food*, Wiley (1995)

Pat Thomas, *Living Dangerously*, Newleaf (2003)

Amanda Ursell, *What are You Really Eating: How to Become Label Savvy*, Hay House (2005)

E. D. Weinberg, *Exposing the Hidden Dangers of Iron*, Cumberland House (2004)

Ruth Winters, *Consumer's Dictionary of Cosmetic Ingredients*, Three Rivers Press (2005)

Ruth Winters, *Consumer's Dictionary of Food Additives*, Three Rivers Press (2009)

Information and a list of relevant books can be obtained from www.price-pottenger.org or by contacting the Price-Pottenger Nutrition Foundation, 7890 Broadway, Lemon Grove, CA 91945, USA. Tel: 00-1-619-462-7600.

Books on detoxing

Kathryn Alexander, *Dietary Healing: The Complete Detox Program*, Annexus (2007)

Stanley Burroughs, *Master Cleanser with Special Needs and Problems*, Stanley Burroughs (1976)

Sandra Cabot, *Liver Cleansing Diet*, Women's Health Advisory Service (WHAS) (1996)

Sandra Cabot and Margaret Jasinska, *Ultimate Detox*, Women's Health Advisory Service (WHAS) (2005)

Bruce Fife, *Detox Book*, Piccadilly Books (2001)

Patrick Holford and Fiona McDonald Joyce, *The Holford 9-Day Liver Detox*, Piatkus (2007)

Bernard Jensen, *Dr Jensen's Guide to Better Bowel Care*, Avery (1999)

Jacqueline Krohn and Frances Taylor, *Natural Detoxification*, Hartley & Marks (2000)

Sidney MacDonald Baker, *Detoxification and Healing*, McGraw-Hill (2003)

Sherry Rogers, *Detoxify or Die*, Prestige Publishing (2002)

Jane Scrivner, *Detox Yourself*, Piatkus (2007)

Norman Walker, *Colon Health*, Norwalk Press (1979)

Brenda Watson, *Detox Strategy*, The Free Press (2008)

Xandria Williams, *Liver Detox Plan*, Vermilion (1988)

Infrared, mobiles and EMFs

Bruce Fife, *Health Hazards of Electromagnetic Radiation*, Piccadilly Books (2009)

David and Ora James, *A Handy Way to Cook Your Brain? Mobile Phones: What's the Damage?*, Body Conservation (2005)

Alasdair and Jean Philips, *The Powerwatch Handbook*, Piatkus (2006)

Cancer

Lise Alschuler and Karolyn Gazella, *Definitive Guide to Cancer*, Celestial Arts (2007)

Ty M. Bollinger, *Step Outside the Box*, Infinity 510 Squared Partners (2006)

Kathleen Deoul, *Cancer Cover Up*, Cassandra Books (2001)

Dr Waltraut Fryda, *Diagnosis Cancer*, Xlibris (2006)

Max Gerson, *A Cancer Therapy*, Totality Books (1958 and 1975)

Burton Goldberg (ed.), *The Alternative Medicine Definitive Guide to Cancer*, Future Medicine Publishing (1997)

James Gordon and Sharon Curtin, *Comprehensive Cancer Care*, Perseus (2000)

Edward Griffin, *World Without Cancer: The Story of Vitamin B_{17}*, American Media (1997)

Lothar Hirnetse, *Chemotherapy Heals Cancer and the World is Flat*, Nexus GmbH (2005)

Josef Issels, *Cancer: A Second Opinion*, G. P. Putnam's Sons (2000)

Ralph Moss, *Cancer Therapy: The Independent Consumer's Guide*, Equinox Press (1993)

Dr David Servan-Schreiber, *Anti Cancer: A New Way Of Life*, Penguin, (2007)

Colin Woollams, *Conventional Cancer Cures, What's the Alternative*, Health Issues (2005)

Lawrence Wilson, *Sauna Therapy*, L.D. Wilson (2006)

Other books by Xandria Williams

Beating the Blues, Vermilion (1999)
Building Stronger Bones, Hamlyn (2002)
Choosing Health Intentionally, Letts Publishing (1992)
Choosing Weight Intentionally, Letts Publishing (1992)
Eating Right: Nutrition, Time-Life Books (1997)
Fatigue: The Secret of Getting Your Energy Back, William Heinemann (1996)
The Four Temperaments, St Martin's Press (1996)
From Stress to Success, Thorsons (2001)
The Herbal Detox Plan, Ebury (2003)
Ideal Weight, Ideal Shape, Wellbeing Golden Keys (2004)
Living with Allergies, Allen and Unwin (1990)
Natural Cures for Common Ailments, Time-Life Books (1997)
Overcoming Candida, Vega (2002)
What's in My Food?, Nature and Health Books (1988)
You're Not Alone, Cedar (1997)

Equipment

Many of the items listed below can be obtained from:
UK Juicers has a wide variety of equipment items. Tel: 01904 757070, www.ukjuicers.com

The Fresh Network sells equipment and a variety of raw foods, such as raw nut butters. Tel: 0845 8337017, www.fresh-network.com

Blenders – heavy duty VitaMix is a high-powered, heavy-duty blender. It will enable you to make many of the foods that are part of the raw food diet. Buy the most powerful you can afford; anything less will soon frustrate you.

Dehydrator Used to dry or 'cook' food below 40ºC (105ºF) and prevent loss of enzymes and valuable nutrients. Square ones with flat trays, such as the Excalibur, have more uses than circular ones with 'walls' around the trays.

Enemas Enema kit with long tubing from Manifest Health. Tel: 01235 838551, www.e-enema.co.uk

Coffee Un-roasted therapeutic enema coffee, such as Wilson brand, available from Manifest Health. Tel: 01235 838551, www.e-enema.co.uk

Far Infra Red (FIR) saunas Get FITT sell a 'sleeping-bag' version, which takes up a minimum of space. Tel: 020 8445 5412, www.get-fitt.com

Juice extractor A heavy-duty screw variety is preferable to the rotating centrifugal basket. These can also be used for making nut butters, humus, etc. Examples include Champion 2000 and Samson. See www.ukjuicers.com and www.fresh-network.com

Sprouting equipment Automatic ones with electrical timer for watering your crop are available. Simpler ones are also available from many health-food shops or some kitchen departments.

Water purification Reverse Osmosis water purifier – this is very much more efficient than a filter, which is only partially and briefly effective. East Midlands Water tel: 0166 276 3334, www.eastmidlandswater.com; The Retreat Company, tel: 0116 259 9211, www.theretreatcompany.com; Fresh Water Company, tel: 0870 4423633, www.freshwaterfilter.com

Laboratories and testing kits

The majority of these laboratories will accept tests only if they have been requested by a practitioner. Their contact details are given here so that you can pass them to your practitioner.

UK

Acumen, John McLaren Howard, P.O. Box 129, Tiverton, Devon EX16 0AJ.
Tel: 07707 877 174, email: acumenlab@hotmail.co.uk
Tests: DNA adducts and other toxins and test for salivary epithelial
growth factor (EGF)

BioLab, Stone House, 9 Weymouth Street, London, W1W 6DB. Tel: 020
7636 5959, www.biolab.co.uk
Tests: a wide range of useful tests, both medical and CAM-appropriate. Ask them for their list

BodyBio Contact via Nutri-Link, Nutrition House, 24 Torquay Road,
Newton Abbott, Devon, TQ12 1AJ. Tel: 01626 882100, 0870 4054 002,
www.nutri-linkltd.co.uk
Tests: computerised analysis of the results of basic blood
biochemistry

BTS Service for the Dr Hauss Laboratory, Germany, in the UK P.O. Box
5279, Brighton, BN50 9DU. Tel: 0844 330 1909
Tests: stool analysis

Doctor's Data (UK office) Tel: 0871 218 0052; elsewhere: 1-630-377-8139,
www.doctorsdata.com
Tests: hair mineral analysis

Genova Diagnostics Europe, Parkgate House, 356 West Barnes Lane, New
Malden, Surrey, KT3 6NB. Tel: 020-8336-7750, email:
infoUK@GDX.net, www.GDX.net
Tests: nearly all the tests for PDFs, in Part One, particularly useful for
CAM-related tests, including the Optimal Nutrition Evaluation, or
ONE, test

Manifold Health Ltd, Oxfordshire, UK. Tel: 01235 838 551, email:
contact@manifesthealth.co.uk, www.manifesthealth.co.uk
Tests: heavy-metal testing kits
Equipment: enema kits and therapeutic coffee for enema use

Neuro Lab Limited, 681 Wimbourne Road, Bournemouth, Dorset, BH9
2AT. Tel: 01202 510 910, email: dntaylor@btconnect.com
Tests: tests for d-lactic acid and l-lactic acid

The Doctor's Laboratory (TDL), 55 Wimpole Street, London. Tel: 020 7307 7383
Tests: a wide range of medical and CAM-appropriate tests

USA

American Metabolic Laboratories, 1818 Sheridan Street, Suite 102, Hollywood, FL 33020. Tel: 001-954-929-4814, www.caprofile.net
Tests: HCG, PHI, CEA, their full CA profile

Analytical Research Laboratories, 2225 W. Alice Avenue, Phoenix, Arizona, 85021 USA. Tel: 001-602-995-1580, www.arltma.com/
Tests: hair analysis and metabolic typing

Doctor's Data Tel: USA: 001-800-323-2784; elsewhere: 001-630-377-8139, www.doctorsdata.com
Tests: hair mineral analysis

Neuroscience Tel: 001-888-342-7272, www.neurorelief.com
Tests: neurotransmitters

Oncolab A free testing kit can be ordered from the USA through the website (www.oncolabinc.com) or by calling: 001-800-922-8378
Test: AMAS test

Trace Element Laboratory, 4501 Sunbelt Drive, Addison, Texas, 75001 USA. Tel: 001-972-250-6410, www.traceelements.com
Tests: hair mineral analysis and metabolic typing

Supplements

Liver Support formulated by Xandria Williams Available in the UK by calling 0-800-212-742, or overseas from 44-1663-718850 or from many health-food shops

AdrenoMax formulated by Xandria Williams is a supplement for adrenal support. It is available from Nutri Imports on 0-800-212-742 (from the UK) or 44-1663-718-850 (elsewhere)

Raw food ideas

The Internet provides a goldmine of information, videos, articles and more that can be perused, downloaded or bought.

Tumour-localised chemotherapy with CAM treatments and information on several German clinics and procedures, www.burtongoldberg.com/index.html

Moss reports and newsletters: www.cancerdecisions.com

Health matters Although many of the resources of this site are US-based, the content matter will help you to understand what to aim for when planning your strategy to regain your health: www.naturalcancer.net/FreeGuide.htm

Kelley's enzyme therapy Click on the picture and listen to the video, click on the book title for details of the therapy. See also William Kelley's book: www.drkelley.com/default.htm, www.drkelley.com, www.whale.to/cancer/k/Contents.html

Dr Gonzalez on enzyme therapy: www.herbtime.com/Information Pages/CancerEnzymeTherapy.htm

Dr Gonzalez on treatment: www.dr-gonzalez.com/history_of_treatment.htm

Budwig protocol: www.alternativehealth.com.au/Articles/ DrBudwigdiet.htm

Dr Fryda's advice: google "Waltraut Fryda cancer". This will lead you to Dr Fryda's excellent book on adrenal exhaustion, lactic acid balancing and cancer

Information on cancer Leads to other sources, including cancer and the immune system: www.keephopealive.org

Metabolic type This website can help you find the diet that is best for you, personally. Click on 'Find Out Your Metabolic Type' then answer the questions. You will be told your metabolic type and given a number of files including a table of nearly all the foods you commonly eat, coloured according to their suitability for you: www.healthexcel.com

Raw food, transitions, recipes, equipment: www.living-foods.com, and www.rawfoodsupport.com

Vegetable recipes For some ideas of a range of vegetable dishes: www.cookitsimply.com. (You will have to filter or modify some of the ingredients.)

Index